MASTER THE™
PHARMACY
TECHNICIAN
CERTIFICATION EXAM (PTCE®)

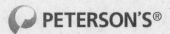 PETERSON'S®

PETERSON'S®

About Peterson's®

Peterson's has been your trusted educational publisher for over 50 years. It's a milestone we're quite proud of, as we continue to offer the most accurate, dependable, high-quality educational content in the field, providing you with everything you need to succeed. No matter where you are on your academic or professional path, you can rely on Peterson's for its books, online information, expert test-prep tools, the most up-to-date education exploration data, and the highest quality career success resources—everything you need to achieve your education goals. For our complete line of products, visit **www.petersons.com.**

For additional information about Peterson's range of educational products, please visit **www.petersons.com**.

Pharmacy Technician Certification Exam®, PTCE®, CPhT™, and PTCB® are all registered trademarks of the Pharmacy Technician Certification Board, which did not collaborate in the production of and does not endorse this product.

For more information, contact Peterson's, 8740 Lucent Blvd., Suite 400, Highlands Ranch, CO 80129, or find us online at **www.petersons.com.**

Peterson's *Master the™ Pharmacy Technician Certification Exam (PTCE®)*

ISBN 978-0-7689-4365-8

Printed in the United States of America

10 9 8 7 6 5 4 3 2   21 20 19

First Edition

Contents

Before You Begin

Peterson's *Master the™ Pharmacy Technician Certification Exam (PTCE®)* gives you the most thorough review and practice available for the Pharmacy Technician Certification Exam. It covers all the domains and knowledge areas tested on the exam, and it gives you the practice you need to earn a high score and gain certification.

WHO SHOULD USE THIS BOOK?

Peterson's *Master the™ Pharmacy Technician Certification Exam (PTCE®)* is written for candidates aiming to pass the Pharmacy Technician Certification Exam (PTCE®), given by the Pharmacy Technician Certification Board (PTCB®). Some states require certification for employment within the profession. Even if your state does not require certification, many employers will look for certification when making their hiring decisions.

This guide is perfect for you if you want a thorough, targeted overview of all domains and knowledge areas tested on the exam alongside test-like practice and detailed feedback.

If you are preparing for your PTCE, use this book if you can answer "yes" to the following statements:

- You want to prepare on your own time and at your own pace, but you don't have time for a preparation program that takes weeks to complete.

- You want a guide that covers all the key points you need to know but doesn't waste time on topics you don't absolutely have to know for the exam.

- You want to avoid taking risks with this all-important exam by relying on "beat the system" guides that are long on promises but short on substance.

- You want a collection of practice tests that look like the exam you will actually take for certification.

HOW THIS BOOK IS ORGANIZED

This book is designed to prepare you to take the PTCE. It's divided into four parts to help you understand the role of the pharmacy technician, the structure of the PTCE, and what you need to know to pass the PTCE and obtain certification. Full-length practice tests are included to help test your knowledge and provide a basis for creating a study plan.

Part I (Chapter 1) gives you a quick overview of the important facts you need to know about the pharmacy technician market, including the ever-changing role of pharmacy technicians in the health care field and the types of jobs available post-certification. You'll also learn all about the PTCE—its use within the industry and question breakdown, and the four main knowledge domains it covers.

Part II (Chapter 2) provides a full-length diagnostic test to help you identify your areas of strength and those areas where you will need to spend more time in your review sessions.

Part III (Chapters 3–6) reviews the topics you need to know to pass the PTCE. The exam is comprised of questions that test your knowledge of the following four knowledge domains:

1. Medications
2. Federal Requirements
3. Patient Safety and Quality Assurance
4. Order Entry and Processing

Part IV (Chapters 7 and 8) contains two full-length practice tests that are as close as you can get to the real thing.

HOW TO USE THIS BOOK

Review **Part I** to familiarize yourself with the pharmacy technician profession and the array of career opportunities. The roles and responsibilities of the technician vary depending upon the industry. This chapter also provides an opportunity to review the structure and content of the PTCE. A sample question for each knowledge domain is shown to illustrate the format of the questions you will encounter.

Take the **Diagnostic Test** in **Part II**. This full-length test is designed to replicate an actual Pharmacy Technician Certification Exam. The questions are aligned with the new test blueprint for 2020. We've provided detailed answer explanations for all answer choices so that you can review why an answer was correct or not correct. Utilize the **Diagnostic Test Assessment Grid** at the end of the chapter to help pinpoint what you know—and what you don't know. Your results provide you with a starting point to tailor your study plan.

Review the chapters in **Part III**. Each chapter covers one knowledge domain in-depth, reviewing all the major concepts you will need to know to pass your exam and gain certification. Before you dive into a chapter, skim the bulleted overview, which lists the topics covered in the lesson. The overview will allow you to quickly target the areas in which you are most interested. At the end of every domain and knowledge area review chapter, you will find 10 practice questions. Use these questions to test your understanding and further assess where you will need to focus your study plan.

Take the practice tests in **Part IV**. Again, the questions align with the percentage of questions from each domain. Take the practice tests under timed conditions and you'll experience just how it feels to take the actual PTCE. As you finish each practice test, check your answers against the answer keys and read the explanation for each question you missed. If you have the time, read all the answer explanations—they're great for even more in-depth PTCE review. You can use your results from these practice tests to see where you need to go back and sharpen your skills before test day.

Print or Online? You Decide!

In addition to the two online tests that are included with the purchase of this book, Peterson's now gives you the option to take the diagnostic and practice tests in Peterson's *Master the*™ *Pharmacy Technician Certification Exam (PTCE®)* either on paper or online. Choose how you want to take them: on paper for a more traditional study approach, or online to simulate the actual PTCE test-taking experience, with automated timing, instant feedback, and scoring results. Take all the tests on paper, all online, or in a combination of the two. The choice is yours.

To access all your free online tests, visit the following URL:
www.petersons.com/testprep/product/pharmacy-technician-online-component/
Add the *PTCE Online Companion* to your cart and enter the coupon code **PHARM1** at checkout.

SPECIAL STUDY FEATURES

Master the™ *Pharmacy Technician Certification Exam (PTCE®)* is designed to be as user-friendly as it is complete. To this end, it includes several features to make your preparation more efficient.

Overview

Each chapter begins with a bulleted overview listing the topics covered in the chapter. This will allow you to quickly target the areas in which you are most interested.

Summing It Up

Each review chapter ends with a point-by-point summary that captures the most important information in the chapter. The summaries are a convenient way to review the main points one last time before the exam.

Notes and Tips

As you make your way through this book, be on the lookout for NOTE and TIP boxes. This bonus information is designed to draw your attention to valuable concepts and test-taking advice, as well as to highlight vital details about the PTCE format.

YOU'RE WELL ON YOUR WAY TO SUCCESS

Congratulations on your new career path! You've made the decision to start a career as a pharmacy technician, and certification is one of the first steps upon your journey. Peterson's *Master the*™ *Pharmacy Technician Certification Exam (PTCE®)* will help you earn a high score and prepare you for everything you'll need to know on the day of your exam and beyond.

Good luck!

GIVE US YOUR FEEDBACK

Peterson's publishes a full line of books—test prep, career preparation, education exploration, and financial aid. Peterson's publications can be found in high school guidance offices, college libraries and career centers, and your local bookstore and library. Peterson's books are also available as eBooks.

We welcome any comments or suggestions you may have about this publication. Your feedback will help us make your education dreams possible for you—and others like you.

PART I
ABOUT THE PHARMACY TECHNICIAN PROFESSION AND CERTIFICATION EXAM

CHAPTER 1   The Pharmacy Technician
            Profession and the PTCE®

The Pharmacy Technician Profession and the PTCE®

OVERVIEW

- The Role of the Pharmacy Technician
- Pharmacy Technician Certification
- The PTCE®
- Summing It Up

THE ROLE OF THE PHARMACY TECHNICIAN

Pharmacy technicians play a vital role in many different areas of pharmacy practice and health care. Opportunities for pharmacy technicians abound—they include working in a variety of areas, including hospital and institutional pharmacies; retail and community practice; mail order, nuclear, infusion and chemotherapy centers; compounding and specialty pharmacies; and even veterinary centers.

Pharmacy technicians have a variety of tasks and responsibilities, based on their location of employment and position within the pharmacy or health care system. In a hospital or institutional pharmacy, a pharmacy technician compounds intravenous (IV) solutions (which may include chemotherapy) and stocks automated dispensing machines for nursing units. Institutional pharmacy technicians are often working in long-term care facilities. The duties of an institutional technician are similar to those in a hospital but may also include filling orders in bubble packs or cards for nursing home residents. In a retail or community pharmacy, pharmacy technicians count medications and resolve insurance issues. Mail order pharmacy technicians communicate with patients, prescribers, and insurance companies and input prescription and insurance information. In a nuclear pharmacy, pharmacy technicians help prepare radiopharmaceuticals to be used for diagnostic testing. A compounding pharmacy technician compounds (or combines) medications in doses or dosage forms that are not commercially available. Veterinary pharmacy technicians specialize in filling prescriptions for animals. Specialty pharmacy technicians, a growing field, may act as care coordinators for patients receiving specialty pharmacy services.

Within each of these locations exists the potential for advancement and growth within the pharmacy technician role. Hospital pharmacy technicians may complete medication reconciliation for patients. Community pharmacy technicians may assist pharmacists in medication therapy management (MTM) or vaccine administration. The pharmacy technician job description continues to evolve and grow as technicians take on more responsibility. As this role continues to expand, many employers or state boards of pharmacy now require certification for pharmacy technicians.

PHARMACY TECHNICIAN TASKS BASED ON HEALTH CARE FACILITY	
Facility	**Pharmacy Technician Duties**
Hospital/Institutional Pharmacy	• Compounds intravenous (IV) solutions • Stocks automated dispensing machines for nursing units • Completes medication reconciliation
Long-Term Care Facility	• Fills orders in bubble packs or cards for nursing home residents
Retail/Community Pharmacy	• Counts medications • Resolves insurance issues • Assists pharmacists in medication therapy management (MTM) • Assists in vaccine administration
Mail-Order Pharmacy	• Communicates with patients, prescribers, and insurance companies • Inputs prescription and insurance information
Nuclear Pharmacy	• Helps prepare radiopharmaceuticals to be used for diagnostic testing
Compounding Pharmacy	• Compounds medications in doses or dosage forms that are not commercially available
Veterinary Pharmacy	• Fills prescriptions for animals
Specialty Pharmacy	• Acts as a care coordinator for patients receiving specialty pharmacy services

PHARMACY TECHNICIAN CERTIFICATION

The Pharmacy Technician Certification Exam (PTCE) is an exam offered by the Pharmacy Technician Certification Board (PTCB). By passing this exam, a pharmacy technician is considered certified, which is a requirement for employment in many states. Once certified, the credentials earned are CPhT—Certified Pharmacy Technician. Two agencies currently offer an exam for pharmacy technician certification: the PTCB and National Healthcareer Association (NHA).

To be certified is not the same as being licensed or registered. A certification is granted by an organization after an individual demonstrates knowledge and skill in a designated area. Some states may also require pharmacy technicians to register with the State Board of Pharmacy, which is essentially enlisting to the state board for tracking and documentation purposes. Additionally, some states may require licensure, which is when the Board of Pharmacy grants permission for practice based on completed requirements or competencies.

> **NOTE**
> The PTCE is recognized in all 50 states, but it is always important to check your state-specific requirements for working as a pharmacy technician.

THE PTCE®

The PTCE consists of 90 questions, of which 80 are scored and 10 are not (these unscored questions are not identified). A total of two hours is allotted for the exam—1 hour and 50 minutes of this time is allowed for the 90 questions, while the remaining 10 minutes is utilized for a beginning tutorial and final survey. To pass the exam, you must earn a score of 1400 (with a range of possible scores of 1000–1600). There is no set number of questions you must answer correctly on your exam; the number differs from test to test depending on the results of all test takers.

Before taking the PTCE, you must fulfill specific eligibility requirements and apply online. The requirements for application include a high school diploma (or GED equivalent or foreign diploma), as well as a full disclosure of any criminal action, which includes Board of Pharmacy registration or licensure issues.

The cost to take the PTCE is $129. Once your application is approved, you have 90 days to take the exam. If you cannot take it within the 90 days, you must withdraw your application, or you may lose your application fee. Because this is a computer-based exam, scheduling can be completed online or by phone and is dependent on your local test center availability.

Starting in 2020, the PTCB will require either completion of a PTCB-recognized education or training program or the equivalent in work experience to qualify to take the PTCE. An attestation form will be completed by pharmacy technician training programs, which will identify if the program meets the standards required to become PTCB-recognized. For experienced working pharmacy technicians who have not completed a PTCB-recognized training program, the technician's employer must also complete an attestation form. This form contains the same knowledge requirements that are used in the PTCB education programs and is used to determine if the work experience gained is equivalent in skills and knowledge that would be obtained in a PTCB-recognized program.

> **NOTE**
>
> Prior to 2020, the PTCE was structured to test nine knowledge domains and areas. Based on a 2016 Job Analysis Study, the exam was restructured into four knowledge domains and areas. For more information, go to the PTCB's website at **www.ptcb.org**.

The Exam Structure

After undergoing a recent evaluation based on a Job Analysis Study, the PTCB restructured the PTCE, removing and adding some of the tested content. As a result, the PTCE now consists of four domains, each one divided into sub-domains or knowledge areas. Each domain has a specific percentage of content allotted for questions on the exam.

Domain	Knowledge Domain	% of PTCE Content	Number of Knowledge Areas
1	Medications	40	10
2	Federal Requirements	12.5	5
3	Patient Safety and Quality Assurance	26.25	6
4	Order Entry and Processing	21.25	5

PTCE® Knowledge Domains

The following is a brief overview of the updated domains and knowledge areas included in each. We've included a sample question for each domain so you can see what it will look like in test format.

Medications

The Medications domain focuses on the components of medications, including over-the-counter (OTC) medications and herbal or dietary supplements. These components include includes generic and brand names, indications (use of a drug to treat a particular disease), interactions, contraindications, side effects, prescribed dosages, and therapy duration. Dosage forms and routes of administration are covered, as well as therapeutic equivalence, proper storage of medications, and common and severe side effects. Medications with narrow therapeutic indexes (NTI) are also included within this domain. With its questions comprising 40% of the exam, the Medications domain makes up the largest portion of the PTCE.

Medications Sample Question

Citalopram can be classified as which class of drug?

A. Antianxiety

B. Antibiotic

C. Antidepressant

D. Antidiabetic

The correct answer is C. Citalopram is an antidepressant.

Federal Requirements

As 12.5% of the exam content, the Federal Requirements domain includes several important regulations and standards that have influenced the practice of pharmacy. These regulations include handling, storing, and disposing of hazardous substances. This domain also includes requirements for the Drug Enforcement Administration (DEA) in regard to controlled substances, such as transferring prescriptions, documentation requirements, and processes for ordering, receiving, returning, and reporting a loss or theft. FDA recall requirements are included in this domain as well as requirements for specific restricted-drug programs.

Federal Requirements Sample Question

A recall that has the potential to cause serious health problems or death is which type?

A. Class I recall

B. Class II recall

C. Class III recall

D. Class IV recall

The correct answer is A. A Class I recall has the potential for serious health problems or death.

Patient Safety and Quality Assurance

Medication safety is an essential component of pharmacy practice. This domain, which is 26.25% of the exam, includes safety strategies, such as understanding error-prone abbreviations and using **tall man lettering**. It also contains look-alike/sound-alike and high-alert or high-risk medications, and error event reporting procedures. In addition, identifying concerns that may necessitate pharmacist intervention is an important area in this domain, as are cleaning standards and hygiene practices, such as cleaning counting trays and hand washing.

> **NOTE**
>
> **Tall man lettering** is the practice used to avoid medication errors by writing part of a medication's name in uppercase letters to differentiate among medications with names that sound alike or look alike. For more information about medication error prevention, see Chapter 5.

Patient Safety and Quality Assurance Sample Question

Which of the following could cause a potential medication error?

- **A.** Leading zero
- **B.** Tall man lettering
- **C.** Trailing zero
- **D.** Bar code scanning

The correct answer is C. A trailing zero can potentially cause a medication error if a dose is misread. For example, 2.0 mg could be misread as 20 mg.

Order Entry and Processing

The Order Entry and Processing domain constitutes 21.25% of the exam. This domain includes processes required when compounding nonsterile products, including calculations known as **alligations**. Also included in this domain is knowledge of lot numbers and expiration dates and understanding National Drug Code (NDC) numbers. Equipment is also part of this domain, which includes supplies needed for drug administration and selecting appropriate package types for each prescription. Calculation knowledge is required to interpret prescriptions; understand abbreviations; and calculate doses, concentration and dilutions, ratios and proportions, and days' supply.

Order Entry and Processing Sample Question

An order is written for 5 mL TID × 10D. How much should be used to fill this prescription?

- **A.** 75 mL
- **B.** 100 mL
- **C.** 150 mL
- **D.** 250 mL

The correct answer is C. 150 mL TID = three times daily. 5 mL × 3 = 15 mL daily. 15 mL × 10 days = 150 mL total.

SUMMING IT UP

- Pharmacy technicians play a vital role in many different areas of pharmacy practice and health care. Career opportunities include working in the following areas:
    - Hospital and institutional pharmacies
    - Long-term care facilities
    - Retail and community practice
    - Mail order pharmacies
    - Nuclear pharmacies
    - Compounding pharmacies
    - Veterinary pharmacies
    - Specialty pharmacies
- Responsibilities and duties vary based on location of employment and position within the pharmacy or health care system.
- Pharmacy technicians must pass an exam to be **certified**. To be certified is not the same as being **licensed** or **registered**. A certification is granted by an organization after an individual demonstrates knowledge and skill in a designated area. Once certified, the credentials earned are **CPhT**.
- Two agencies offer an exam for certification—the **Pharmacy Technician Certification Board (PTCB)** and the **National Healthcareer Association (NHA)**.
- The **Pharmacy Technician Certification Exam (PTCE)** is offered by the PTCB. The exam consists of 90 questions, of which 80 are scored and 10 are not. The 10 unscored questions are not identified.
- A total of two hours is allotted to take the PTCE—1 hour and 50 minutes for 90 questions, and 10 minutes for the beginning tutorial and final survey.
- The cost to take the PTCE is $129. Applicants must fulfill specific eligibility requirements and apply online. Once the application is approved, individuals have 90 days to take the exam.
- Since the PTCE is a computer-based exam, scheduling can be completed online or by phone and is dependent upon local test center availability.
- The PTCE is structured into four knowledge domains:
    1. Medications
    2. Federal Requirements
    3. Patient Safety and Quality Assurance
    4. Order Entry and Processing

- The **Medications** domain comprises 40% of the exam, making it the largest portion of the PTCE. This knowledge domain focuses on the following:
  - Generic and brand names of medications
  - Over-the-counter (OTC) medications and herbal or dietary supplements
  - Indications (the use of a drug to treat a particular disease)
  - Interactions
  - Contraindications
  - Common and severe side effects
  - Prescribed dosages, dosage forms, and routes of administration
  - Therapy duration
  - Proper storage

- The **Federal Requirements** domain comprises 12.5% of the PTCE, and includes important regulations and standards that have influenced the practice of pharmacy. Questions in this knowledge domain include the following:
  - Handling, storing, and disposing of hazardous substances
  - Drug Enforcement Administration (DEA) requirements for controlled substances
    - Transferring prescriptions
    - Documentation requirements
    - Ordering, receiving, and returning processes
    - Reporting a loss or theft
  - FDA recall requirements
  - Restricted-drug program requirements

- The **Patient Safety and Quality Assurance** domain comprises 26.25% of the PTCE, and includes the following:
  - Medication safety
  - Error-prone abbreviations
  - Look-alike/sound-alike (LASA) medications
  - High-alert/high-risk medications
  - Error prevention and reporting
  - Cleaning standards and hygiene practices

- The **Order Entry and Processing** domain constitutes 21.25% of the exam. Questions in this knowledge domain test the following:
  - Processes for compounding non-sterile products
  - Lots numbers and expiration dates
  - National Drug Code (NDC) numbers
  - Equipment and supplies needed for drug administration
  - Appropriate prescription package types
  - Calculation knowledge is required to interpret prescriptions, understand abbreviations, and calculate the following:
    - Doses
    - Concentration and dilutions
    - Ratio and proportions
    - Days' supply

PART II
DIAGNOSING YOUR STRENGTHS AND WEAKNESSES

CHAPTER 2   Diagnostic Test

ANSWER SHEET DIAGNOSTIC TEST

1. Ⓐ Ⓑ Ⓒ Ⓓ	19. Ⓐ Ⓑ Ⓒ Ⓓ	37. Ⓐ Ⓑ Ⓒ Ⓓ	55. Ⓐ Ⓑ Ⓒ Ⓓ	73. Ⓐ Ⓑ Ⓒ Ⓓ
2. Ⓐ Ⓑ Ⓒ Ⓓ	20. Ⓐ Ⓑ Ⓒ Ⓓ	38. Ⓐ Ⓑ Ⓒ Ⓓ	56. Ⓐ Ⓑ Ⓒ Ⓓ	74. Ⓐ Ⓑ Ⓒ Ⓓ
3. Ⓐ Ⓑ Ⓒ Ⓓ	21. Ⓐ Ⓑ Ⓒ Ⓓ	39. Ⓐ Ⓑ Ⓒ Ⓓ	57. Ⓐ Ⓑ Ⓒ Ⓓ	75. Ⓐ Ⓑ Ⓒ Ⓓ
4. Ⓐ Ⓑ Ⓒ Ⓓ	22. Ⓐ Ⓑ Ⓒ Ⓓ	40. Ⓐ Ⓑ Ⓒ Ⓓ	58. Ⓐ Ⓑ Ⓒ Ⓓ	76. Ⓐ Ⓑ Ⓒ Ⓓ
5. Ⓐ Ⓑ Ⓒ Ⓓ	23. Ⓐ Ⓑ Ⓒ Ⓓ	41. Ⓐ Ⓑ Ⓒ Ⓓ	59. Ⓐ Ⓑ Ⓒ Ⓓ	77. Ⓐ Ⓑ Ⓒ Ⓓ
6. Ⓐ Ⓑ Ⓒ Ⓓ	24. Ⓐ Ⓑ Ⓒ Ⓓ	42. Ⓐ Ⓑ Ⓒ Ⓓ	60. Ⓐ Ⓑ Ⓒ Ⓓ	78. Ⓐ Ⓑ Ⓒ Ⓓ
7. Ⓐ Ⓑ Ⓒ Ⓓ	25. Ⓐ Ⓑ Ⓒ Ⓓ	43. Ⓐ Ⓑ Ⓒ Ⓓ	61. Ⓐ Ⓑ Ⓒ Ⓓ	79. Ⓐ Ⓑ Ⓒ Ⓓ
8. Ⓐ Ⓑ Ⓒ Ⓓ	26. Ⓐ Ⓑ Ⓒ Ⓓ	44. Ⓐ Ⓑ Ⓒ Ⓓ	62. Ⓐ Ⓑ Ⓒ Ⓓ	80. Ⓐ Ⓑ Ⓒ Ⓓ
9. Ⓐ Ⓑ Ⓒ Ⓓ	27. Ⓐ Ⓑ Ⓒ Ⓓ	45. Ⓐ Ⓑ Ⓒ Ⓓ	63. Ⓐ Ⓑ Ⓒ Ⓓ	81. Ⓐ Ⓑ Ⓒ Ⓓ
10. Ⓐ Ⓑ Ⓒ Ⓓ	28. Ⓐ Ⓑ Ⓒ Ⓓ	46. Ⓐ Ⓑ Ⓒ Ⓓ	64. Ⓐ Ⓑ Ⓒ Ⓓ	82. Ⓐ Ⓑ Ⓒ Ⓓ
11. Ⓐ Ⓑ Ⓒ Ⓓ	29. Ⓐ Ⓑ Ⓒ Ⓓ	47. Ⓐ Ⓑ Ⓒ Ⓓ	65. Ⓐ Ⓑ Ⓒ Ⓓ	83. Ⓐ Ⓑ Ⓒ Ⓓ
12. Ⓐ Ⓑ Ⓒ Ⓓ	30. Ⓐ Ⓑ Ⓒ Ⓓ	48. Ⓐ Ⓑ Ⓒ Ⓓ	66. Ⓐ Ⓑ Ⓒ Ⓓ	84. Ⓐ Ⓑ Ⓒ Ⓓ
13. Ⓐ Ⓑ Ⓒ Ⓓ	31. Ⓐ Ⓑ Ⓒ Ⓓ	49. Ⓐ Ⓑ Ⓒ Ⓓ	67. Ⓐ Ⓑ Ⓒ Ⓓ	85. Ⓐ Ⓑ Ⓒ Ⓓ
14. Ⓐ Ⓑ Ⓒ Ⓓ	32. Ⓐ Ⓑ Ⓒ Ⓓ	50. Ⓐ Ⓑ Ⓒ Ⓓ	68. Ⓐ Ⓑ Ⓒ Ⓓ	86. Ⓐ Ⓑ Ⓒ Ⓓ
15. Ⓐ Ⓑ Ⓒ Ⓓ	33. Ⓐ Ⓑ Ⓒ Ⓓ	51. Ⓐ Ⓑ Ⓒ Ⓓ	69. Ⓐ Ⓑ Ⓒ Ⓓ	87. Ⓐ Ⓑ Ⓒ Ⓓ
16. Ⓐ Ⓑ Ⓒ Ⓓ	34. Ⓐ Ⓑ Ⓒ Ⓓ	52. Ⓐ Ⓑ Ⓒ Ⓓ	70. Ⓐ Ⓑ Ⓒ Ⓓ	88. Ⓐ Ⓑ Ⓒ Ⓓ
17. Ⓐ Ⓑ Ⓒ Ⓓ	35. Ⓐ Ⓑ Ⓒ Ⓓ	53. Ⓐ Ⓑ Ⓒ Ⓓ	71. Ⓐ Ⓑ Ⓒ Ⓓ	89. Ⓐ Ⓑ Ⓒ Ⓓ
18. Ⓐ Ⓑ Ⓒ Ⓓ	36. Ⓐ Ⓑ Ⓒ Ⓓ	54. Ⓐ Ⓑ Ⓒ Ⓓ	72. Ⓐ Ⓑ Ⓒ Ⓓ	90. Ⓐ Ⓑ Ⓒ Ⓓ

Answer Sheet

Diagnostic Test

90 Questions—110 minutes

> **Directions:** This diagnostic test is designed to help you recognize your strengths and weaknesses. The questions cover information across the four knowledge domains presented on the PTCE®. For each of the following items, choose the correct answer and then fill in the corresponding circle on the answer sheet. Check your answers using the answer key and explanations that follow the test, and then use the assessment grid to focus your study plan.

1. A pharmacy becomes aware of a Class 1 recall for a specific lot number of diabetic test strips. Which of the following should occur?
   A. The pharmacy can continue to dispense the strips, as a Class 1 recall does not cause patient harm.
   B. The pharmacy must quarantine the strips immediately, as a Class 1 recall can cause adverse events or death.
   C. The pharmacy can dispense the strips and inform patients of the recall so they can make their own decision.
   D. The pharmacy can monitor usage and sales to determine if any patients have an adverse event.

2. The generic name for Neurontin is
   A. pregabalin.
   B. albuterol.
   C. cyclobenzaprine.
   D. gabapentin.

3. Which medication is classified as high-alert, due to the potential for serious tissue injury if infiltrated during IV administration?
   A. Meclizine
   B. Promethazine
   C. Ondansetron
   D. Prochlorperazine

4. Which of the following should be avoided by patients taking spironolactone?
   A. Salt substitutes
   B. Dairy products
   C. Orange juice
   D. Chocolate

5. The SDS for a drug will give which of the following information?
   A. Dosing guidelines
   B. Drug interactions
   C. Handling and storage information
   D. Diluent to be used for reconstitution

6. A 22-pound child is to receive a prescription for Augmentin dosed as 30 mg/kg/day q12h. If the pharmacy stocks a 250 mg/5 mL suspension, how many mL are given for each dose?
   A. 2.5 mL
   B. 3 mL
   C. 4 mL
   D. 6 mL

7. Which of the following is a beta blocker?
   A. Rosuvastatin
   B. Atenolol
   C. Clonazepam
   D. Losartan

8. Which of the following is true regarding the ordering of Schedule II medications?

   A. A technician may order Schedule II medications using a wholesaler account.

   B. A pharmacist can order using CSOS or DEA Form 222.

   C. A duplicate form can be completed by the technician for ordering.

   D. A pharmacist can assign a technician to be a delegate for ordering Schedule II medications.

9. Which of the following dosages must be clarified before dispensing?

   A. 0.5 mg

   B. 0.005 mg

   C. 5 mcg

   D. 5.0 mcg

10. A patient requests assistance in finding something OTC to help with her arthritis. What supplement would the pharmacist recommend?

    A. St. John's wort

    B. Echinacea

    C. Cranberry

    D. Glucosamine

11. A patient is attempting to purchase three boxes of pseudoephedrine. Each box contains 1.7 grams. Can the pharmacy technician sell this quantity to the patient?

    A. Yes, this is under the daily limit of 7.5 grams.

    B. No, this exceeds the daily limit of 2.4 grams.

    C. No, this exceeds the daily limit of 3.6 grams.

    D. Yes, there is no daily limit, only a limit for 30 days.

12. Which of the following suffixes indicate a drug is an ACE inhibitor?

    A. –olol

    B. –pril

    C. –artan

    D. –cillin

13. A patient tells a pharmacy technician that she is feeling miserable and needs an OTC cold medication. The patient mentions that she is on a medication for high blood pressure and asks if this is a problem. Which would be the best response from the pharmacy technician?

    A. There is no interaction with high blood pressure. You can find the cough and cold medications in aisle 5.

    B. The pharmacist should help you with this question. I will bring him over for a consultation.

    C. You cannot take cold medication while on high blood pressure medication. You should consult your physician to change medications.

    D. Taking an OTC vitamin would be better suited for you if you have high blood pressure. This will be much safer.

14. A patient brings in a prescription on Sunday evening for oxycodone 5 mg. The pharmacy does not have the full amount to fill the entire prescription. When must the remaining quantity be available for the patient?

    A. By Wednesday evening

    B. By the following Sunday evening

    C. By 30 days from the date of first filling

    D. A partial fill is not allowed.

15. Which of the following medications is taken as one weekly dose of 70 mg?

    A. Alendronate

    B. Metformin

    C. Diltiazem

    D. Buproprion

16. Interpret the following prescription order:
    1 TAB PO TID AC PRN HA

    A. Take 1 tablet by mouth twice daily after meals as needed for heartburn.

    B. Take 1 tablet by mouth three times daily before meals as needed for headache.

    C. Take 1 tablet by mouth twice daily before meals as needed for high blood pressure.

    D. Take 1 tablet by mouth three times daily as needed for headache.

17. Which type of error is one that is caught before reaching the patient?

    A. Omission

    B. Near miss

    C. Administration

    D. Ordering

18. Which of the following OTC medications is an antihistamine?

    A. Pseudoephedrine

    B. Loratadine

    C. Dextromethorphan

    D. Guaifenesin

19. A device attached to an inhaler, to make it easier for children to breathe in the medication (sometimes with a mask), is a(n)

    A. spacer.

    B. nebulizer.

    C. MDI.

    D. atomizer.

20. After counting which of the following medication should the counting tray be cleaned with 70% IPA?

    A. Sulfamethoxazole with trimethoprim

    B. Lovastatin

    C. Aspirin

    D. Accupril

21. iPledge is a REMS program for which medication?

    A. Entereg

    B. Isotretinoin

    C. Mycophenolate

    D. Nplate

22. The DEA form required for theft of controlled substances is

    A. DEA Form 41.

    B. DEA Form 106.

    C. DEA Form 222.

    D. DEA Form 224.

23. Certification for laminar air flow hoods or isolator glove boxes must occur how often?

    A. Every 30 days

    B. Every 3 months

    C. Every 6 months

    D. Every year

24. Each day, a pharmacy technician reviews prescriptions that have not been picked up. As per the pharmacy policy, after 10 days of sitting in the will-call bin, these medications are then

    A. disposed of in the pharmaceutical waste.

    B. left for another 30–60 days for patients to pick up.

    C. returned to stock.

    D. segregated and quarantined.

25. Meloxicam belongs to which drug classification?

    A. Potassium-sparing diuretic

    B. Anticoagulant

    C. NSAID

    D. Antiepileptic

26. A reverse distributor is a third party who returns expired medications to manufacturers and wholesalers for

    A. a one-to-one replacement.

    B. credit.

    C. a fee.

    D. other pharmacies to buy at a discount.

Diagnostic Test

27. The USP chapter that defines non-sterile compounding standards is
    A. 795.
    B. 797.
    C. 800.
    D. 825.

28. Preventing, monitoring, and managing the potential hazards of a medication's use by providing education to the patient and health care provider is known as
    A. quarantining.
    B. reverse distribution.
    C. risk evaluation and mitigation strategies.
    D. prescribing authority.

29. Which of the following medications should be taken at bedtime?
    A. Lovastatin
    B. Levothyroxine
    C. Hydrochlorothiazide
    D. Furosemide

30. What is the first step in donning PPE before compounding sterile products?
    A. Putting on shoe covers
    B. Putting on sterile gloves
    C. Putting on a sterile gown
    D. Putting on a mask

31. Which of the following is an inactive ingredient or "filler" used in a compound with an active medication?
    A. Phospholipid
    B. PLO gel
    C. Aliquot
    D. Excipient

32. Zofran ODT is administered
    A. intramuscularly.
    B. subcutaneously.
    C. orally on the tongue.
    D. rubbed on the skin.

33. A pharmacy dispenses Wellbutrin XL to a patient with the instructions to take TID. Which type of prescription error would this be?
    A. Incorrect quantity
    B. Incorrect patient
    C. Incorrect dosing
    D. Incorrect concentration

34. Which temperature range would be appropriate for the storage of latanoprost?
    A. 20°C to 25°C
    B. 80°F to 95°F
    C. −25°F to −10°F
    D. 2°C to 8°C

35. Which of the following drugs is a high-alert medication?
    A. Amlodipine
    B. Cephalexin
    C. Epinephrine
    D. Sertraline

36. A patient has a prescription for 20 grams of hydrocortisone cream 10%. The pharmacy has 2% and 20% in stock. How much of each is required to compound this prescription?
    A. 5 grams of 2% and 15 grams of 20%
    B. 8 grams of 2% and 12 grams of 20%
    C. 11 grams of 2% and 9 grams of 20%
    D. 12 grams of 2% and 8 grams of 20%

37. A prescription for alprazolam could be refilled a maximum of
    A. 0 times; no refills are permitted.
    B. 3 times within 30 days.
    C. 5 times within 6 months.
    D. 12 times within one year.

38. What is the purpose of tall man lettering?

    A. To identify specific strengths of medications

    B. To differentiate dosage forms of the same medication

    C. To clarify NDC numbers in the computer system

    D. To distinguish between look-alike/sound-alike medications

39. A patient calls and asks how long her insulin will last before she must discard it. She says she used the first dose on March 3. Which date would the pharmacy technician tell the patient she should discard the insulin?

    A. March 10

    B. March 17

    C. March 28

    D. March 31

40. What does the final set of numbers indicate on an NDC?

    A. Manufacturer

    B. Drug

    C. Package size

    D. Expiration date

41. A process that helps identify any factors involved in a medication error or adverse event is known as a

    A. continuous quality improvement.

    B. drug utilization review.

    C. medication use evaluation.

    D. root cause analysis.

42. Which of the following dosage forms should be avoided by diabetic patients?

    A. Liniment

    B. Enema

    C. Syrup

    D. Suspension

43. What is the generic name for Lantus?

    A. Insulin detemir

    B. Insulin glargine

    C. Insulin aspart

    D. Insulin lispro

44. Which of the following is NOT a primary route of infectious disease transmission?

    A. Contact

    B. Droplet

    C. Pandemic

    D. Airborne

45. Which needle type must be used to remove fluid from an ampule?

    A. Hypodermic

    B. Insulin

    C. Filter

    D. Transfer

46. Which of the following must be avoided while taking metronidazole?

    A. Grapefruit juice

    B. Milk

    C. Alcohol

    D. Diet soda

47. Discoloration of urine is a side effect of which medication?

    A. Nitrofurantoin

    B. Liraglutide

    C. Timolol

    D. Acyclovir

48. A patient receives 30 tablets of alprazolam with the instructions, take 1 PO TID PRN anxiety. The patient returns for a refill after 7 days because she is out of medication. Which of the following prescription errors would this be?

    A. Early refill

    B. Incorrect quantity

    C. Incorrect patient

    D. Wrong drug

Diagnostic Test

49. What is the proper procedure for disposing of non-hazardous pharmaceutical waste?

    A. Liquid medications are discarded in the sink, and solid tablets or capsules are flushed down the toilet.

    B. All medications, regardless of dosage form, are rinsed down the sink.

    C. It should be sorted in a segregated container and incinerated.

    D. It should be disposed of with the bio-hazard waste.

50. The packaging (bottle or unit dose) for which of the following medications is also considered hazardous due to potential residue?

    A. Albuterol

    B. Warfarin

    C. Cephalexin

    D. Losartan

51. A pediatric patient has a prescription for amoxicillin suspension with a dose of 125 mg q8hr × 7d. The pharmacy gives the patient an 80 mL bottle of suspension (125 mg/5 mL), and counsels the mother to make sure to take it until it's gone to ensure the entire antibiotic therapy is completed. This would be which type of prescription error?

    A. Abnormal doses

    B. Early refill

    C. Incorrect quantity

    D. Incorrect drug

52. Which of the following tools used for blood sugar monitoring consists of a sharp needle used to prick the skin?

    A. Glucometer

    B. Lancet

    C. Test strip

    D. Insulin needle

53. When two drugs contain the same active ingredient and dosage and utilize the same route of administration and meet all the same standards for purity and quality, they are known as

    A. therapeutically equivalent.

    B. agonists.

    C. pharmacokinetics.

    D. antagonists.

54. Invoices of Schedule II controlled substances, as well as completed CSOS or 222 forms, must be stored in the pharmacy (or a secured off-site location) for how many years?

    A. 2 years

    B. 5 years

    C. 7 years

    D. 10 years

55. The FDA system used to report adverse medication events is

    A. VAERS.

    B. MedWatch.

    C. ISMP.

    D. OBRA.

56. An example of a medication in which a small difference in dosage may lead to a serious adverse event or insufficient therapeutic response would be

    A. atorvastatin.

    B. lisinopril.

    C. warfarin.

    D. amoxicillin.

57. A pharmacy technician fills a prescription for a liquid with a total volume of 110 mL. Which package size should be selected for dispensing?

    A. 2 fl. oz.

    B. 3 fl. oz.

    C. 4 fl. oz.

    D. 6 fl. oz.

58. Which of the following medications is indicated for symptomatic treatment of BPH (Benign prostatic hyperplasia)?
    A. Meclizine
    B. Levofloxacin
    C. Gemfibrozil
    D. Terazosin

59. Which error prevention technique is often found on patient wrist bands and drug packaging, and is verified prior to prescription dispensing or administration of a medication?
    A. Separating inventory
    B. Tall man lettering
    C. Bar code scanning
    D. Leading zeroes

60. A solid dosage form, inserted into the rectum, vagina, or urethra is a(n)
    A. emulsion.
    B. enema.
    C. suppository.
    D. capsule.

61. After reconstitution, azithromycin can be used for how many days before it must be discarded?
    A. 5 days
    B. 10 days
    C. 14 days
    D. 21 days

62. A pharmacy technician is entering a prescription into a patient's profile. After submitting the order, an alert appears with information the pharmacist needs to verify. The process of identifying and reviewing problems, such as drug allergies, doses that are too high, or contraindication is known as
    A. therapeutic substitution (TS).
    B. drug utilization review (DUR).
    C. continuous quality improvement (CQI).
    D. root cause analysis (RCA).

63. The generic name for Xarelto is
    A. apixaban.
    B. dabigatran.
    C. rivaroxaban.
    D. clopidogrel.

64. Which capsule size listed is the largest?
    A. 000
    B. 0
    C. 1
    D. 5

65. Which of the following drugs, if taken with ciprofloxacin, may cause a serious drug interaction and risk of bleeding?
    A. Warfarin
    B. Pregabalin
    C. Oxcarbazepine
    D. Irbesartan

66. Which of the following is the process of mixing drugs into a compound by adding the smallest ingredient first, then mixing evenly the same amount as the next ingredient, and repeating steps until all amounts have been mixed (to provide an even distribution throughout the compound)?
    A. Trituration
    B. Levigation
    C. Spatulation
    D. Geometric dilution

67. A patient with asthma would want to avoid which medication for treatment of high blood pressure?
    A. Enalapril
    B. Losartan
    C. Metoprolol
    D. Diltiazem

68. A patient takes Nexium 20 mg at home. This patient is admitted to the hospital, and Nexium is not on the hospital formulary, so the pharmacist converts the order to Prilosec 20 mg. This is an example of
    A. incorrect drug medication error.
    B. medication adherence.
    C. therapeutic substitution.
    D. drug utilization review.

69. Which of the following routes of administration would be instilled into the ear?
    A. Buccal
    B. Ophthalmic
    C. Sublingual
    D. Otic

70. Which of the following would be used in the event of a recall to identify the specific medication recalled?
    A. Expiration date
    B. Unit dose
    C. Lot number
    D. Wholesaler

71. Which of the following medications must be taken until the duration of drug therapy is complete?
    A. Docusate
    B. Ondansetron
    C. Doxycycline
    D. Naproxen

72. Which of the following medications may cause a patient to have a persistent cough?
    A. Propranalol
    B. Ramipril
    C. Clonazepam
    D. Zolpidem

73. A medication that has the month/year as the expiration date, expires on the
    A. 1st day of the month.
    B. 7th day of the month.
    C. 15th of the month.
    D. last day of the month.

74. Which of the following medications should be stored in its original container to protect from light sensitivity?
    A. Nitroglycerin
    B. Paroxetine
    C. Allopurinol
    D. Loratidine

75. Which of the following medications must be stored in a safe or locked cabinet at all times?
    A. Simvastatin
    B. Escitalopram
    C. Pseudoephedrine
    D. Oxycodone

76. A pharmacy receives a prescription for cyclobenzaprine 10 mg 1 TID PRN #30. What would be the days' supply for this prescription?
    A. 7 days
    B. 10 days
    C. 15 days
    D. 30 days

77. The abbreviation "HS" intended to mean at bedtime, is often misinterpreted as
    A. hours.
    B. hold syringe.
    C. sufficient quantity.
    D. half-strength.

78. A pharmacy technician is compounding the components of two capsules together with a diluent. She notices that the color of the mixture changes suddenly to a dark brown. This would be an example of
    A. chemical incompatibility.
    B. physical incompatibility.
    C. levigation incompatibility.
    D. reconstitution incompatibility.

79. Ginkgo biloba may be used to treat which of the following?
    A. Blood pressure
    B. Menopausal symptoms
    C. Memory and dementia
    D. Fatigue

80. Taking levofloxacin could result in which of the following adverse effects?
    A. Hypernatremia
    B. Tendonitis or rupture
    C. Rectal bleeding
    D. Hypoglycemia

81. Which medication should not be taken with acetaminophen or a product containing acetaminophen (for example, cold and flu medication)?
    A. Advil
    B. Oxycontin
    C. Morphine
    D. Percocet

82. Tyramine, a component in some cheeses, can cause a serious interaction with which drug?
    A. Escitalopram
    B. Selegiline
    C. Amitriptyline
    D. Paroxetine

83. Which drug is considered a high-alert medication?
    A. Lantus
    B. Predinsone
    C. Toradol
    D. Singulair

84. A patient weighs 82 pounds and has an order for a medication to take 4 mg/kg daily. The medication is available in several different strengths. Which of the following would be closest for the patient's dose?
    A. 75 mg tablet
    B. 150 mg tablet
    C. 300 mg tablet
    D. 500 mg tablet

85. Risperidone is in which class of medications?
    A. COX-2 inhibitor
    B. Sulfonylurea
    C. Antifungal
    D. Antipsychotic

86. Which of the following must be included with prescriptions for specific medications which have been determined that certain information is necessary to prevent adverse events?
    A. Black box warning
    B. Product package insert
    C. Medication guide
    D. Privacy statement

87. A patient has a sulfa allergy. Which medication must be avoided?
    A. Omnicef
    B. Amoxil
    C. Bactrim
    D. Abilify

Diagnostic Test

88. How many mg of lidocaine are needed to prepare 25 mL of a 1% lidocaine solution?

    A. 0.25 mg

    B. 5 mg

    C. 50 mg

    D. 250 mg

89. A patient has stated that he often misses doses of his prescription for metoprolol, because it makes him tired and he doesn't like to feel sleepy. The pharmacist must consult this patient regarding

    A. adherence.

    B. allergies.

    C. therapeutic substitution.

    D. OTC recommendation.

90. Which medication is often taken as a tapered dosage, to allow the adrenal glands time to resume normal function?

    A. Diphenhydramine

    B. Sumatriptan

    C. Nifedipine

    D. Prednisone

ANSWER KEY AND EXPLANATIONS

1. B	16. B	31. D	46. C	61. B	76. B
2. D	17. B	32. C	47. A	62. B	77. D
3. B	18. B	33. C	48. A	63. C	78. B
4. A	19. A	34. D	49. C	64. A	79. C
5. C	20. A	35. C	50. B	65. A	80. B
6. B	21. B	36. C	51. C	66. D	81. D
7. B	22. B	37. C	52. B	67. C	82. B
8. B	23. C	38. D	53. A	68. C	83. A
9. D	24. C	39. D	54. A	69. D	84. B
10. D	25. C	40. C	55. B	70. C	85. D
11. C	26. B	41. D	56. C	71. C	86. C
12. B	27. A	42. C	57. C	72. B	87. C
13. B	28. C	43. B	58. D	73. D	88. D
14. A	29. A	44. C	59. C	74. A	89. A
15. A	30. A	45. C	60. C	75. D	90. D

1. **The correct answer is B.** The pharmacy must quarantine the strips immediately, as a Class 1 recall can cause adverse events or death. In a Class 1 recall, there is a reasonable probability that the use of the recalled product will cause serious adverse health consequences or death. The pharmacy must not continue to dispense the strips (choice A) or allow the patient to make their own choice on using (choice C). Monitoring usage and sales in anticipation of potential adverse events (choice D) would not be the correct action to take.

2. **The correct answer is D.** Gabapentin is the generic name for Neurontin. Pregabalin (choice A) is the generic name for Lyrica. Albuterol (choice B) is the generic name for Proventil. Cyclobenzaprine (choice C) is the generic name for Flexeril.

3. **The correct answer is B.** Promethazine (Phenergan) IV can cause serious caustic tissue damage if infiltrated during IV administration. Meclizine, ondansetron, and prochlorperazine are all medications used for antinausea, but are not considered high-alert.

4. **The correct answer is A.** Patients taking spironolactone must avoid salt substitutes and foods with a high potassium content. Dairy products, orange juice, and chocolate are safe to eat while taking spironolactone.

5. **The correct answer is C.** The SDS provides information on chemicals considered hazardous, including properties of the chemical, safe handling and storage practices, and how to treat exposure. Choices A and D are incorrect because dosing guidelines and diluents used for reconstitution would be included with a package insert. Drug interactions (choice B) would be found in a pharmacy reference such as Lexicomp.

6. **The correct answer is B.** The first step is to convert the patient's weight from lbs. to kg.

Answers Diagnostic Test

$$\frac{22 \text{ lbs.}}{2.2} = 10 \text{ kg}$$

So 30 mg × 10 kg = a dose of 300 mg/day. Now calculate mL:

$$\frac{x \text{ mL}}{300 \text{ mg}} = \frac{5 \text{ mL}}{250 \text{ mg}}$$

$$x = 6 \text{ mL}$$

The daily dose is 6 mL.
For each dose (q12h), divide by 2.
Thus 6 ÷ 2 = 3 mL per dose.

7. **The correct answer is B.** Atenolol is a beta blocker. Rosuvastatin (choice A) is a statin, clonazepam (choice C) is a benzodiazepine, and losartan (choice D) is an ARB (angiotensin II receptor blocker).

8. **The correct answer is B.** A pharmacist can order using CSOS or DEA Form 222. Schedule II medications can be ordered only by a pharmacist through CSOS or DEA Form 222. A technician cannot order Schedule II medications but is permitted to order Schedule III–V medications. DEA Form 222 is a triplicate form, not duplicate, and cannot be completed by a technician. A pharmacist is not permitted to assign a delegate for ordering Schedule II medications.

9. **The correct answer is D.** The dosage 5.0 mcg has a trailing zero and should be clarified before dispensing. The trailing zero is dangerous because it can be confused or misread as 50 mcg. Choice C (5 mcg) demonstrates how this dosage should be written. Dosages 0.5 mg (choice A) and 0.005 mg (choice B) are both safe with leading zeroes.

10. **The correct answer is D.** Glucosamine may help reduce arthritis-related pain and relieve joint swelling and pain. St. John's wort (choice A) is used for mild depression. Echinacea (choice B) helps reduce symptoms of colds and to promote the immune system. Cranberry (choice C) is used for urinary tract health or urinary tract infections.

11. **The correct answer is C.** The pharmacy technician cannot sell this quantity to the patient. Three boxes of 1.7 grams

pseudoephedrine equals 5.1 grams, which exceeds the daily limit of 3.6 grams.

12. **The correct answer is B.** ACE inhibitors all end in *–pril* (e.g., lisinopril or enalapril). Beta blockers end in *–olol*, ARBs end in *–artan*, and pencillin antibiotics end in *–cillin*.

13. **The correct answer is B.** The best response would be for the pharmacy technician to tell the patient that the pharmacist should help with this question and then bring the pharmacist to the patient for a consultation. The other answer options are incorrect because it is out of the scope of practice for a pharmacy technician to answer clinical questions regarding OTC selection and potential interaction with a prescription medication. There is interaction with certain cold medications and raising blood pressure, but the pharmacist can review with the patient the need to consult a physician and possibly change a prescription. Vitamins may help treat the cold, but there are some that may interact with medications as well, and they are not always the safer option.

14. **The correct answer is A.** A Schedule II medication can be partially filled if the remaining quantity is provided within 72 hours. If additional quantities are required after 72 hours, a new prescription must be written by the provider.

15. **The correct answer is A.** Alendronate, used to treat osteoporosis, is taken as a weekly dose. Metformin (choice B) is taken once or twice daily. Diltiazem (choice C) may be dosed up to four times daily. Buproprion (choice D) is taken daily.

16. **The correct answer is B.** The definitions in this sig code are as follows:
TAB = tablet
PO = by mouth
TID = three times daily
AC = before meals
PRN = as needed
HA = headache
Combining all of these abbreviations translates to: Take 1 tablet by mouth three times daily before meals as needed for headache.

17. **The correct answer is B.** A near miss occurs when an error is caught before it can reach or harm the patient. Near misses are an essential component to an error-reporting program, as these often indicate an unsafe trend or pattern of almost-errors. An omission error (choice A) results when a medication error occurs due to an omission, such as missing a patient's scheduled dose administration. Administration errors (choice C) occur when there is an error during drug delivery, such as a medication intended for use in the eye getting administered into the ear. An ordering error (choice D) occurs when a provider is entering an order and a mistake is made and not caught prior to administering the incorrect order.

18. **The correct answer is B.** Loratadine is an antihistamine. Pseudoephedrine (choice A) is a decongestant. Dextromethorphan (choice C) is a cough suppressant. Guaifenesin (choice D) is an expectorant.

19. **The correct answer is A.** A spacer is a tube that attaches to an inhaler and keeps the medication enclosed in order for a child to breathe in more easily. A nebulizer (choice B) is a machine that turns a liquid medication into a mist to be inhaled. An MDI (choice C) is a metered dose inhaler that regulates a dose of medication, such as albuterol, with each puff. An atomizer (choice D) turns a liquid medication into a mist (similar to a nebulizer) but is smaller in size, such as one used to administer nasally.

20. **The correct answer is A.** A counting tray should be cleaned with 70% IPA after counting sulfamethoxazole with trimethoprim. This medication is a sulfa, and residue from the tablets can remain on the counting tray after counting. Cleaning with 70% IPA will prevent cross-contamination of any powder or residue to another patient's tablets or capsules. The other answer choices are incorrect because lovastatin, aspirin, and accupril are not medications to which patients have a hypersensitivity or allergy.

21. **The correct answer is B.** iPledge is a program for isotretinoin (Accutane, Clarivis) that permits only patients who meet all the qualifications of the program to take isotretinoin. Due to the extreme potential for birth defects if a patient were to become pregnant, this program includes agreeing to two forms of birth control as well as two negative pregnancy tests prior to receiving the prescription. A female patient must continue to take monthly pregnancy tests before refilling the prescription. Entereg (choice A) is a REMS to prevent myocardial infarction requiring use for short-term only. The mycophenolate REMS (choice C) is related to a high potential for miscarriage and risk of birth defects. The Nplate REMS (choice D) is to inform patients and health care workers of the potential for bone marrow fibrosis and worsened thrombocytopenia.

22. **The correct answer is B.** DEA Form 106 must be completed electronically or on an original paper copy to submit to the DEA. DEA Form 41 (choice A) is used for destruction of outdated or damaged controlled substances. DEA Form 222 (choice C) is used for ordering Schedule II substances. A DEA Form 224 (choice D) is required for a pharmacy to be registered with the DEA.

23. **The correct answer is C.** Hoods must be certified to be compliant with USP Chapter <797> standards every 6 months.

24. **The correct answer is C.** A pharmacy technician reviews the medications hanging in the pickup area each day for those that have been on the shelf for a designated (per pharmacy) time period. After this time, the medication is removed from the prescription bag and returned to the stock shelf to be dispensed to another patient. The medication does not need to be disposed of (choice A). Medications should not be left for 30–60 days (choice B), as this would impact insurance billing as well as expiration dating. The medications do not need to be segregated or quarantined (choice D) and can be dispensed to other patients.

Answers Diagnostic Test

25. **The correct answer is C.** Meloxicam is an NSAID. Potassium-sparing diuretics (choice A) are used for hypertension and congestive heart failure. Anticoagulants (choice B) inhibit the clotting of blood. An antiepileptic (choice D) controls the symptoms of epilepsy.

26. **The correct answer is B.** A reverse distributor returns expired or unusable medications to manufacturers on behalf of a pharmacy and gives the pharmacy credit based on what items are returned. Choices A and C are incorrect because reverse distributors do not replace medications, and the fee is removed from the credit owed the pharmacy. Choice D is incorrect because other pharmacies cannot purchase expired drugs for a discount.

27. **The correct answer is A.** USP <795> is the chapter which defines standards for non-sterile compounding. USP <797> (choice B) addresses standards related to sterile compounding. USP <800> (choice C) outlines standards for hazardous drugs and workplace safety. USP <825> (choice D) addresses standards for compounding radiopharmaceuticals.

28. **The correct answer is C.** Risk evaluation and mitigation strategies (REMS) are used to evaluate risks of using drugs considered dangerous by the FDA. Without these strategies, such medications would either be removed from the market or be denied FDA approval. Quarantining (choice A) would be done if a recalled medication needed to be removed from stock. Reverse distribution (choice B) most often refers to a company or vendor who is registered with the DEA to receive controlled substances from another pharmacy and process them (return to manufacturer or arrange for disposal). A prescribing authority (choice D) is someone who has the authorization or license to write prescriptions.

29. **The correct answer is A.** Statins, such as Lovastatin, should be taken right before bedtime, as most cholesterol is produced during sleep. Levothyroxine (choice B)

should be taken in the morning. Hydrochlorothiazide (choice C) and furosemide (choice D) are both diuretics and, if taken at bedtime, could cause the patient to have to urinate during the night.

30. **The correct answer is A.** The first step in donning PPE before entering the clean room is to put on shoe covers. This keeps any potential contamination on the shoes out of the clean room. Choices B, C, and D all occur after putting on shoe covers. The next step of PPE garbing would be to put on a mask. After hands are washed and cleaned, the technician can put on a sterile gown. Finally, the technician enters the clean room and uses an alcohol-based cleanser prior to putting on sterile gloves.

31. **The correct answer is D.** An excipient is an inert substance used in non-sterile compounding. A phospholipid (choice A) is part of the cell membrane. PLO gel (choice B) is a type of compound used transdermally. An aliquot (choice C) is a small portion of a substance.

32. **The correct answer is C.** ODT stands for orally disintegrating tablet. Zofran ODT is administered orally to dissolve on the tongue. The terms *intamuscularly* (choice A) and *subcutaneously* (choice B) both refer to injections. Rubbing on the skin (choice D) would be a transdermal route of administration.

33. **The correct answer is C.** A patient taking Wellbutrin XL (and most medications that are a controlled release formulation) does not take the medication three times daily because the controlled release formulation is designed to last longer. An incorrect quantity error (choice A) would be dispensing the wrong number of units of a medication, such as giving 30 tablets for a prescription that called for 60 tablets. The incorrect patient error (choice B) occurs when a prescription is filled under the wrong profile. An incorrect concentration error (choice D) would occur if a suspension was reconstituted and too much or too little diluents were added.

34. **The correct answer is D.** Latanoprost must be stored in the refrigerator, and the storage range for refrigerated medications is between 2°C and 8°C. Choice A is room temperature storage range. Choice B is generally too warm (above room temperature) for medication storage. Choice C is the wrong temperature scale.

35. **The correct answer is C.** Epinephrine is on the high-alert medication list, due to the risk of harm to patients given the wrong dose or when given in error. Amlodipine, cephalexin, and sertraline are not on the high-alert medication list.

36. **The correct answer is C.** To solve, use the alligation method:

    Step 1: Place the desired strength in the middle (10%).

    Step 2: Place the higher strength in stock on the top left corner.

    Step 3: Place the lower strength in stock in the bottom left corner.

    Step 4: Subtract the middle strength from the top left and place in the bottom right corner.

    Step 5: Subtract the bottom left strength from the middle and place in the top right corner.

    Step 6: Add up the right column to get the total parts needed.

    Step 7: Set up ratios to determine how much of each stock strength is needed. Use the totals in the right column for each strength.

20		8
	10	
2		10
		18 total parts

For the 2% hydrocortisone cream:

$$\frac{10 \text{ parts}}{18 \text{ parts}} = \frac{x \text{ grams}}{20 \text{ grams}}$$
$$(10)(20) = 18x$$
$$\frac{200}{18} = x$$
$$x \approx 11 \text{ grams}$$

For the 20% hydrocortisone cream:

$$\frac{8 \text{ parts}}{18 \text{ parts}} = \frac{x \text{ grams}}{20 \text{ grams}}$$
$$(8)(20) = 18x$$
$$\frac{160}{18} = x$$
$$x \approx 9 \text{ grams}$$

37. **The correct answer is C.** Alprazolam is a Schedule IV controlled substance and cannot be filled more than 5 times within 6 months. Schedule II controlled substances are not permitted to have refills.

38. **The correct answer is D.** Tall man lettering helps emphasize the parts of a drug name, distinguish between look-alike/sound-alike medications, and help prevent medication errors. The other answer choices are incorrect because tall man lettering does not identify medication strengths or dosage forms, and it does not represent a specific NDC number.

39. **The correct answer is D.** Once opened, a vial of insulin must be discarded after 28 days, which in this case, is March 31. Choices A, B, and C are too early; March 10 is 10 days, March 17 is 14 days, and March 28 is 25 days.

40. **The correct answer is C.** The final set of numbers of an NDC is the package size. The first set of numbers is the labeler code and assigned by the FDA. The labeler is the manufacturer (choice A) or vendor of the medication. The second set of numbers, which identifies the drug (choice B) and strength, is the product code. The expiration date (choice D) is not in the NDC number format.

Answers Diagnostic Test

41. **The correct answer is D.** A root cause analysis (RCA) is a process completed in response to an adverse medication event that helps identify any workflows, practices, or procedures that may have contributed to the event. Choice A is incorrect because continuous quality improvement (CQI) is a management process that promotes ongoing improvement procedures. Choice B is incorrect because drug utilization review (DUR) is a review of patient prescription information before receiving a medication. Choice C is incorrect because a medication use evaluation (MUE) is conducted to determine if appropriate prescribing and usage patterns exist for high cost, error prone, or specific medications.

42. **The correct answer is C.** A syrup is a liquid dosage form containing sugar that could disrupt the blood sugar of a diabetic patient. A liniment (choice A) is an emulsion applied through rubbing of the skin. An enema (choice B) is a solution administered rectally. A suspension (choice D) is a two-part liquid and powder system that does not dissolve.

43. **The correct answer is B.** The generic name of Lantus is insulin glargine. Insulin detemir (choice A) is the generic for Levemir. Insulin aspart (choice C) is the generic for Novolog. Insulin lispro (choice D) is generic for Humalog.

44. **The correct answer is C.** A pandemic is an outbreak of a disease, such as influenza. It is not a primary route of infectious disease transmission. Contact, droplet, and airborne are all primary routes of infectious disease transmission. Contact transmission (choice A) occurs when direct or indirect contact is made with an infected individual. Droplets (choice B) are transmitted through sneezing, coughing, or talking. Airborne disease (choice D) is transferred through small particles suspended in the air.

45. **The correct answer is C.** A filter needle must be used when compounding using an ampule, as the needle is designed to filter any particulates or glass shards to prevent from contaminating the final solution. A hypodermic needle (choice A) is the needle type used for most sterile compounds. Insulin syringes (choice B) are small, 1 mL syringes that are used for insulin (they are measured in units). A transfer needle (choice D) is two needles that are attached at the hub to transfer solutions from one vial to another.

46. **The correct answer is C.** If a patient consumes alcohol while taking metronidazole (Flagyl), serious abdominal cramps, nausea, vomiting, and headaches can occur. Metronidazole does not interact with grapefruit juice, milk, or diet soda.

47. **The correct answer is A.** Nitrofurantoin causes the urine to turn a rust or brown color. Liraglutide, timolol, and acyclovir do not cause urine discoloration.

48. **The correct answer is A.** The patient's directions were to take 1 tablet three times daily as needed and dispense 30 tabs. With these directions, the patient should have enough to last a maximum of 10 days. If the patient is out after 7 days, this is an early refill and the patient is most likely taking the prescription inappropriately. Choices B and C are incorrect because the correct quantity was dispensed, and it was given to the correct patient. Choice D is incorrect because the correct drug was given—alprazolam is indicated for treatment of anxiety.

49. **The correct answer is C.** Non-hazardous pharmaceutical waste is discarded in a designated disposal method and collected to be incinerated. Choices A and B are incorrect because medications should not be flushed down the toilet or in the sink. Choice D is incorrect because biohazard waste should not include pharmaceutical waste.

50. **The correct answer is B.** Due to the anticoagulating properties of warfarin, the packaging must also be treated as hazardous and disposed as such because it may contain

residue. Albuterol, cephalexin, and losartan are all exempt from this requirement.

51. **The correct answer is C.** The patient is taking 125 mg/5 mL q8h = 3 times daily. 5 mL × 3 = 15 mL daily × 7d = 105 mL total needed for this therapy. The pharmacy dispenses an 80 mL bottle, which will not be a sufficient quantity for the patient to complete the antibiotic therapy. The dose is not abnormal (choice A), and the patient is not getting a refill (choice B). Choice D is incorrect because the drug is filled as written.

52. **The correct answer is B.** A lancet is a small needle encased in plastic that pricks the finger to draw blood for testing. A glucometer (choice A) is a device that uses blood to calculate the blood glucose level. A test strip (choice C) is used to collect the blood from the finger after the lancet has pierced the skin. An insulin needle (choice D) is used to administer insulin.

53. **The correct answer is A.** Therapeutically equivalent drugs must be bioequivalent (have the same response at the same rate), be of the same dosage form, and contain the same active ingredient and route of administration. An agonist (choice B) is a medication or substance that turns on or initiates a response at a receptor. Pharmacokinetics (choice C) is the study of absorption, distribution, metabolism and elimination (ADME) properties of a drug in the body. An antagonist (choice D) is a medication or substance that inhibits or blocks a receptor or inhibits an action.

54. **The correct answer is A.** All invoices and ordering records for Schedule II controlled substances must be stored for two years. Schedule III–V medications may be ordered by any method, and invoices must also be stored for two years. These must be separate from non-controlled invoices.

55. **The correct answer is B.** The FDA utilizes MedWatch as an online voluntary reporting system for adverse medication events. VAERS (choice A) is the Vaccine Adverse Event Reporting System. ISMP (choice C) is the Institute for Safe Medication Practices, which establishes guidelines for medication safety. OBRA (choice D) is the Omnibus Budget Reconciliation Act, which requires pharmacists to counsel and perform a drug utilization review on each patient.

56. **The correct answer is C.** A drug with a narrow therapeutic index is one in which a small difference in dosage may lead to a serious adverse event or insufficient therapeutic response. Warfarin is an anticoagulant, and too high of a dose could cause bleeding, whereas too small of a dose could cause a blood clot. Atorvastatin (choice A) is used for cholesterol, lisinopril (choice B) is used for blood pressure, and amoxicillin (choice D) is an antibiotic. These drugs do not have a narrow therapeutic index.

57. **The correct answer is C.** 1 fl. oz. is equal to 30 mL, so 4 fl. oz. is equal to 120 mL. When selecting package size, it's important to get as close to the volume as possible, without overfill. Choices A and C are incorrect because 2 fl. oz. would be 60 mL, and 3 fl. oz. would be 90 mL; neither size would be big enough for 120 mL. Choice D is incorrect because 6 fl. oz. would be 180 mL, which would be too big.

58. **The correct answer is D.** Terazosin is indicated for treatment of symptomatic BPH. Meclizine (choice A) is indicated for treatment of nausea and vomiting. Levofloxacin (choice B) is used for treatment of bacterial infections, including community-acquired pneumonia or UTI. Gemfibrozil (choice C) is used to help reduce LDL or bad cholesterol and triglycerides in the body.

59. **The correct answer is C.** Bar codes are found on drug packaging and patient wrist bands. These are scanned prior to administering medications in an institutional facility. Bar codes are also placed on drug packaging and are scanned prior to prescription dispensing in a pharmacy. Separating inventory (choice A) helps prevent errors when selecting products and verifying that

the correct drug is selected. Tall man lettering (choice B) is used to help identify specific medications that look alike. Leading zeroes (choice D) are used to prevent dosing errors with oral liquid medications.

60. **The correct answer is C.** A solid dosage form (at room temperature) that is inserted rectally, vaginally, or urethrally is a suppository. Upon insertion into the body, the suppository will melt, and the medication is then released. An emulsion (choice A) is a stabilized mixture of oil and water that does not separate. An enema (choice B) is a liquid that is administered into the rectum. A capsule (choice D) is a solid dosage form used most frequently to take by mouth.

61. **The correct answer is B.** Azithromycin suspension has a shelf life after reconstitution of 10 days. Choice A is incorrect because at 5 days, the suspension is still good for administration. Choices C and D are incorrect because the medication will no longer be stable at 14 and 21 days, respectively.

62. **The correct answer is B.** A drug utilization review (DUR) is completed prior to submitting to any insurance company and utilizes the computer system to identify any potential issues with the patient's prescription. Therapeutic substitution (choice A) occurs when a medication prescribed is exchanged or substituted with another medication determined to have the same clinical effect. CQI (choice C) is continuous ongoing improvement, and an RCA (choice D) is completed as an investigation following a major error or event.

63. **The correct answer is C.** Xarelto is the name brand for rivaroxaban. Apixaban (choice A) is the generic for Eliquis, dabigatran (choice B) is the generic for Pradaxa, and clopidogrel (choice D) is the generic for Plavix.

64. **The correct answer is A.** For capsules, the smaller the number, the larger the capsule. In this case, the largest to smallest capsule sizes are 000, then 0, 1, and 5.

65. **The correct answer is A.** Ciprofloxacin increases the activity of warfarin, which can cause bleeding if the warfarin dosage is not adjusted during ciprofloxacin therapy. Pregabalin, oxcarbazepine, and irbesartan (choices B, C, and D, respectively) do not interact with ciprofloxacin.

66. **The correct answer is D.** Geometric dilution is the process of mixing an active drug into a compound by adding the smallest ingredient first, and then evenly adding the same amount of another ingredient, until all ingredients have been mixed. Trituration (choice A) is the process of reducing the size of particles by grinding. Levigation (choice B) is combining a powder and a liquid (such as an ointment). Spatulation (choice C) is combining a mixture by mixing them together using a spatula.

67. **The correct answer is C.** Metoprolol is a beta blocker, and this class of drugs can interact with the beta receptors that are used for treatment with bronchodilators for asthma treatment. Enalapril (choice A) is an ACE inhibitor, losartan (choice B) is an ARB, and diltiazem (choice D) is a calcium channel blocker—these drug classes do not interact with beta receptors.

68. **The correct answer is C.** Therapeutic substation (also known as therapeutic interchange) occurs when a medication is substituted for another within the same drug class that has the same clinical effects. This would not be considered a medication error (choice A). Medication adherence (choice B) is taking medications correctly, and drug utilization review (choice D) utilizes the computer system to identify any potential issues with the patient's prescription.

69. **The correct answer is D.** The otic route of administration refers to medication put into the ear. A buccal administration (choice A) occurs by placement in the cheek, an ophthalmic administration (choice B) is instilled into the eye, and a sublingual administration (choice C) is placed under the tongue.

70. **The correct answer is C.** The lot number is a unique identifier that corresponds to a particular batch of medication manufactured. This identifier helps track lots of medication that may be impacted by a recall when other lots are not. The expiration date (choice A), unit dose information (choice B), and wholesaler (choice D) are not needed in a recall.

71. **The correct answer is C.** Doxycycline is an antibiotic, and completing the entire course of therapy is essential to prevent antibiotic resistance and the infection returning. Docusate (choice A) is used for constipation and can be taken as needed. Ondansetron (choice B) is used for nausea and vomiting, and it can be taken when symptoms occur. Naproxen (choice D) is an NSAID, is used for inflammation and pain relief, and can also be taken as needed.

72. **The correct answer is B.** Ramipril is an ACE inhibitor, and this class of medications can cause patients to have a cough as a side effect. Propranalol (choice A) is a beta blocker and does not have coughing as a side effect. Clonazepam (choice C) is a benzodiazepine, and zolpidem (choice D) is a hypnotic—neither of these drug classes cause a cough to occur as a side effect.

73. **The correct answer is D.** A medication that has only a month and year expiration date (for example 9/2021) would expire on the last day of September in the year listed. That means it will be good through the entire month before expiration.

74. **The correct answer is A.** Nitroglycerin tablets must be stored in their original container, an amber vial, to protect from degradation of the medication due to light sensitivity. Paroxetine, allopurinol, and loratidine do not require light-resistant packaging and can be counted and placed in a medication vial.

75. **The correct answer is D.** Oxycodone is a Schedule II medication and must therefore be kept in locked storage. Simvastatin (choice A) and escitalopram (choice B) are not controlled substances and do not require

additional security for storage. Pseudo-ephedrine (choice C) is an OTC item that must be stored behind the counter, but it does not require locked storage.

76. **The correct answer is B.** The directions would read, 1 tablet three times daily as needed. The patient could take a maximum of 3 tablets daily, and the total quantity dispensed is 30 tablets.

$$\frac{30 \text{ tab}}{3 \text{ tab per day}} = 10 \text{ days}$$

77. **The correct answer is D.** "HS" is on the ISMP list of error-prone abbreviations because it is often misinterpreted as half-strength. While this abbreviation should not be used, pharmacy technicians may still encounter its use in pharmacy practice. Choice A is incorrect because the abbreviation for *hours* is "hr." or "hrs." *Hold syringe* (choice B) is not typically abbreviated, and *sufficient quantity* (choice C) is abbreviated as "QS."

78. **The correct answer is B.** Physical incompatibility occurs when a reaction between two or more substances causes a change in color, odor, taste, or viscosity. A chemical incompatibility (choice A) occurs when a reaction causes a change in the chemical properties of the compound. Levigation (choice C) is the process of triturating a powder drug with a solvent. Reconstitution (choice D) is the process of adding a diluent to a powder to form a solution or suspension.

79. **The correct answer is C.** Ginkgo biloba is often used to improve memory and prevent dementia. Choice A is incorrect because fish oil is a supplement used for blood pressure. Choice B is incorrect because soy is used to treat symptoms of menopause. Choice D is incorrect because ginseng can be used for fatigue and chronic fatigue syndrome.

80. **The correct answer is B.** Levofloxacin is a flouroquinolone antibiotic, and this drug class has a black box warning for the potential of tendonitis or tendon rupture. The other answer choices are incorrect because hypernatremia (high blood sodium), rectal

bleeding, and hypoglycemia (low blood sugar) are not side effects of levofloxacin.

81. **The correct answer is D.** Percocet is a combination narcotic analgesic, which includes acetaminophen and oxycodone. If a patient is taking Percocet, there is the potential for liver damage if additional acetaminophen is taken in excess of four grams per day. Choice A is incorrect because Advil and acetaminophen are often taken together in alternating doses for fever or pain relief. Choices B and C are incorrect because oxycontin (oxycodone) and morphine do not contain acetaminophen.

82. **The correct answer is B.** Selegiline is an MAOI, and eating tyramine while taking a medication in this class can cause a major hypertensive emergency. Escitalopram (choice A) and paroxetine (choice D) are SSRIs, and amitryiptyline (choice C) is a tricyclic antidepressant. These drugs do not interact with tyramine.

83. **The correct answer is A.** Lantus is an insulin medication and all insulins are considered high-alert medications. Prednisone, Toradol (ketorolac), and Singulair (montelukast) are not high-alert medications.

84. **The correct answer is B.** The weight must first be converted from lbs. into kg.

$$\frac{82.5 \text{ lbs.}}{2.2} = 37.3 \text{ kg}$$

Next, multiply the per day dose by the total kg.

4 mg × 37.3 kg = 149.2 mg

The dose is then rounded to the closest package size, which would be 150 mg.

85. **The correct answer is D.** Risperidone is used to treat mental or mood disorders and is classified as an antipsychotic. An example of a COX-2 inhibitor (choice A) would be celecoxib. An example of a sulfonylurea (choice B) is glipizide, and terbinafine is an example of an antifungal medication (choice C).

86. **The correct answer is C.** A medication guide must be distributed with specific medications the FDA has determined need additional detailed information to

prevent adverse events. A black box warning (choice A) is applied to a drug when there is evidence the drug may cause serious harm. A product package insert (choice B) is packaged with each drug and includes technical information for pharmacy or medical staff. The privacy statement (choice D) must be displayed or presented upon request for patient privacy information.

87. **The correct answer is C.** A patient allergic to sulfa would have a reaction to Bactrim (sulfamethoxazole and trimethoprim). Omnicef (choice A) is a cephalosporin antibiotic, and Amoxil (choice B) is a penicillin antibiotic. Abilify (choice D) is an antipsychotic used to treat mood disorders.

88. **The correct answer is D.** The 1% solution is a w/v so 1 gram in 100 mL. To calculate how many mg of lidocaine are needed for 25 mL of the 1% solution, set up a ratio proportion:

$$\frac{1 \text{ gram}}{100 \text{ mL}} = \frac{x \text{ gram}}{25 \text{ mL}}$$

Then solve for x:

$$\frac{25}{100} = .25 \text{ grams}$$

Convert the grams to mg:

0.25 g × 1,000 = 250 mg

89. **The correct answer is A.** Adherence is taking a medication as prescribed. It can be very dangerous for a patient to miss doses or not take the medication as the provider intended. Allergies, therapeutic substitution, and OTC recommendations are all important pharmacist consultation areas, but not required for missing doses and adherence.

90. **The correct answer is D.** Prednisone is a steroid used to suppress the immune system to help treat allergic reactions, skin conditions, arthritis, or lupus. Prednisone dosing must be tapered, or reduced slowly, to allow the adrenal glands time to resume normal function. Diphenhydramine (choice A) is an antihistamine, sumatriptan (choice B) is a triptan used to treat migraines, and nifedipine (choice C) is a calcium channel blocker.

DIAGNOSTIC TEST ASSESSMENT GRID

Now that you've completed the diagnostic test and read through the answer explanations, you can use your results to target your studying. The following table shows you exactly where you can find thorough coverage for each knowledge domain. Find the question numbers from the diagnostic test that gave you the most trouble and highlight or circle them below. The chapters with the most markings are your ideal starting points on your preparation journey.

Knowledge Domain	Question Number	Chapter Reference
Medications	2, 4, 7, 10, 12, 15, 18, 25, 29, 32, 34, 39, 42, 43, 46, 47, 53, 56, 58, 61, 63, 65, 67, 69, 71, 72, 74, 75, 78–82, 85, 87, 90	Chapter 3
Federal Requirements	1, 5, 8, 11, 14, 21, 22, 28, 37, 49, 50, 54	Chapter 4
Patient Safety and Quality Assurance	3, 9, 13, 17, 20, 23, 27, 33, 35, 38, 41, 44, 48, 51, 55, 59, 62, 68, 77, 83, 86, 89	Chapter 5
Order Entry and Processing	6, 16, 19, 24, 26, 30, 31, 36, 40, 45, 52, 57, 60, 64, 66, 70, 73, 76, 84, 88	Chapter 6

What question type gave you the most trouble?

- ❑ Medications
- ❑ Federal Requirements
- ❑ Patient Safety and Quality Assurance
- ❑ Order Entry and Processing

Chapters to focus on first: _____

PART III
PTCE® REVIEW

Medications

OVERVIEW

- **Generic Names, Brand Names, and Classifications of Medications**
- **Common and Life-Threatening Drug Interactions and Contraindications**
- **Strengths/Dose, Dosage Forms, Routes of Administration, Special Handling and Administration Instructions, and Duration of Drug Therapy**
- **Common and Severe Medication Side Effects, Adverse Effects, and Allergies**
- **Indications of Medications and Dietary Supplements**
- **Narrow Therapeutic Index (NTI) Medications**
- **Physical and Chemical Incompatibilities Related to Non-Sterile Compounding and Reconstitution**
- **Proper Storage of Medications**
- **Summing It Up**
- **Practice Questions: Medications**
- **Answer Key and Explanations**

An understanding of basic pharmacology is important when learning about drug classes, interactions, and a drug's effect on the body. **Pharmacology** is the study of the uses, effects, and mechanism of action of drugs. Within pharmacology are two branches of study, known as pharmacodynamics and pharmacokinetics. **Pharmacodynamics** is the study of the effects of a drug on the body, while **pharmacokinetics** examines the movement of a drug within the body during the absorption, distribution, metabolism, and elimination or excretion (ADME) processes.

Absorption, the first phase of a medication action, is the process of a drug entering the bloodstream. Next, the drug is distributed **(distribution)** from the blood to tissues and cells throughout the body. **Metabolism**, the process of breaking down or converting the drug into a form that is more easily excreted, is next. The final step, **elimination**, is the process of drug removal from the body.

It is important to have an understanding of each phase of this process, as each phase will impact drug action. For example, medications delivered intravenously work more quickly than those taken by mouth because an IV medication is injected directly into the bloodstream, while medications taken by mouth must be first digested in the stomach before absorption into the bloodstream. Routes of administration and dosage forms, therefore, have an impact on absorption.

Distribution is dependent upon the tissues or cells that a drug affects. If a drug activates a receptor in a cell to initiate a response, it is known as an **agonist**. If it blocks the receptor or binds without activating, it is known as an **antagonist**.

Once a drug has been distributed, enzymes are used to **metabolize**, or break down, the drug into components that can be eliminated. Many drug interactions occur due to effects on enzymatic response. If an enzyme is induced, it will metabolize a drug more rapidly, causing less of an effect or lower quantity of drug to be in the blood. If an enzyme is blocked, the drug will not be metabolized, and may be at toxic levels or create unwanted side effects. The liver is the primary location of drug metabolism.

Elimination of most medications occurs through the kidneys. Some drugs may also be excreted through sweat, tears, saliva, or even breast milk. When a patient has renal impairment, elimination or renal clearance may be impacted. This may cause a modification in dosing to prevent toxicity or accumulation of a metabolized drug.

GENERIC NAMES, BRAND NAMES, AND CLASSIFICATIONS OF MEDICATIONS

The Food and Drug Administration (FDA) must approve all drugs before they are introduced to the public. This approval ensures that the drug is both safe and effective. When a drug is approved by the FDA, it has three names: the chemical name, generic name, and brand name. The **chemical name** of a drug is a complex description of the molecular structure and is generally not used. Instead, the pharmaceutical company that created the drug will market its use under a brand name.

The **generic name** of a drug is assigned by the United States Adopted Names (USAN) Council. The USAN Council utilizes a nomenclature (naming) process to assign generic drug names that help identify drug action, specifically in the stem of the name. For example, beta blockers all end in *–olol*. This naming process begins when a drug is undergoing clinical trials, and the drug end action and class may be determined.

The **brand name**, also known as the trade or proprietary name, is created by the drug company. The FDA must approve all brand names, and it must be distinct from the generic name. While the generic name follows a naming convention and is often a form of the chemical name, brand names tend to be more memorable or catchy, and sometimes describe the purpose of the drug. For example, Flomax is a medication used to treat enlarged prostate and help urine flow. This helps prescribers and patients remember names more easily.

Brand name medications are protected by a patent for a period of time. This allows the developing drug company to sell the drug exclusively until the patent expiration. With no generic competition, a patent allows for the recoup of research and development expenses for the new drug. Once the patent has expired, the generic version of the drug can be produced by another company or manufacturer (after FDA approval). Generic drugs can be sold for a lower price because the manufacturer does not have to spend the time and money on research and clinical trials. The FDA approval process for generic drugs is generally less time-consuming than that for brand name drugs because it requires the submission of the shortened Abbreviated New Drug Application (ANDA), rather than a New Drug Application (NDA). Before approval, the FDA requires the generic drug manufacturer to demonstrate equivalence in dosage form, strength, and route of administration to the brand name medication. The generic drug must also meet the same safety and quality standards as the brand name drug and, as a result, work the same as the brand name medication.

Below are the chemical and generic names for Tylenol.

Chemical Name	N-(4-hydroxyphenyl) acetamide
Generic Name	Acetaminophen
Brand Name	Tylenol

A **drug class** is a group of medications that are similar either in structure, mechanism of action, or in the disease or condition they are used to treat. Generic drugs that are in the same class will often end or begin with the same stem.

The following table lists drug stems and the drug classes associated with each. Although this is not a comprehensive list, it can help identify a majority of the most commonly prescribed drugs and their classes.

Drug Stem	Drug Class	Drug Examples
-azepam	Antianxiety—Benzodiazepine	Lorazepam (Ativan)
-azosin	Antihypertensive—Alpha blocker	Terazosin (Hytrin)
-caine	Local anesthetic	Lidocaine (Xylocaine)
Cef-	Antibiotic—Cephalosporins	Cefazolin (Kefzol)
-cillin	Antibiotic—Penicillins	Amoxicillin (Amoxil)
-conazole	Antifungal—Systemic	Fluconazole (Diflucan)
-curium, -curonium	Neuromuscular blocker	Mivacurium (Mivacron) Rocuronium (Zemuron)
Estr-	Estrogens	Estradiol (Estrace)
-etanide	Diuretic—Loop	Bumetanide (Bumex)
-fibrate	Antihyperlipidemic	Fenofibrate (Tricor)
-gliptin	Oral hypoglycemic—DPP4 inhibitor	Sitagliptin (Januvia)
-lukast	Antiasthmatic/Antiallergy	Montelukast (Singulair)
-mab	Monoclonal antibodies	Adalimumab (Humira)
-micin	Antibiotic	Gentamicin (Garamycin)
-mycin	Antibiotic	Vancomycin (Vancocin)
-olol	Beta blocker	Metoprolol (Lopressor)
-olone	Corticosteroid	Prednisolone (Orapred)
-oxacin	Antibiotic—Fluoroquinolone	Ciprofloxacin (Cipro)
-pezil	Alzheimer's treatment	Donepezil (Aricept)
-pidem	Hypnotic	Zolpidem (Ambien)
-platin	Antineoplastic	Cisplatin (Platinol)
-prazole	Antiulcer	Lansoprazole (Prevacid)
-pril	ACE inhibitor	Lisinopril (Prinivil)
-profen	Anti-inflammatory agents	Ibuprofen (Motrin)
-sartan	Antihypertensive—Angiotensin II receptor blocker (ARB)	Losartan (Cozaar)
-semide	Diuretic—Loop	Furosemide (Lasix)
-setron	Serotonin receptor antagonist	Ondansetron (Zofran)
-statin	Antihyperlipidemic—HMGCoA reductase inhibitor	Atorvastatin (Lipitor)

Drug Stem	Drug Class	Drug Examples
Sulfa-	Antimicrobial—Sulfonamide	Sulfamethoxazole/trimethoprim (Bactrim)
-terol	Bronchodilator	Albuterol (Proventil)
-thiazide	Diuretic—Thiazide	Hydrochlorothiazide (HydroDiuril)
-tidine	H2 receptor antagonist	Ranitidine (Zantac)
-toin	Antiepileptic	Phenytoin (Dilantin)
-triptan	Antimigrane agent	Sumatriptan (Imitrex)
-triptyline	Antidepressant—Tricyclic	Amitriptyline (Elavil)
-vir	Antiviral	Oseltamivir (Tamiflu)

As a pharmacy technician, it is important to understand and remember brand, generic, and drug classes for the most commonly prescribed medications. Below is a list of commonly prescribed medications and their drug class for your review.

Generic Name	Brand Name	Drug Class
Acetaminophen	Tylenol	Analgesic
Acyclovir	Zovirax	Antiviral
Adalimumab	Humira	Monoclonal antibody
Albuterol	Proventil	Bronchodilator
Albuterol sulfate with ipratropium bromide	Combivent, Duoneb	Combination bronchodilator
Alendronate	Fosamax	Bisphosphonate
Allopurinol	Zyloprim	Antigout
Alprazolam	Xanax	Antianxiety—Benzodiazepine
Amiodarone	Cordarone	Antiarrhythmic
Amitriptyline	Elavil	Antidepressant—Tricyclic
Amlodipine	Norvasc	Antihypertensive—Calcium channel blocker
Amlodipine with benazepril	Lotrel	Antihypertensive—Combination agent
Amoxicillin	Amoxil	Antibiotic—Penicillin
Amoxicillin with clavulanate	Augmentin	Antibiotic—Penicillin
Apixaban	Eliquis	Direct oral anticoagulants (DOAC)

Generic Name	Brand Name	Drug Class
Aripiprazole	Abilify	Antipsychotic
Aspirin	Ecotrin	Antipyretic, Analgesic
Atenolol	Tenormin	Antihypertensive—Beta blocker
Atorvastatin	Lipitor	Antihyperlipidemic—HMG-CoA reductase inhibitor
Azithromycin	Zithromax	Antibiotic—Macrolide
Bacitracin, neomycin, polymyxin B	Neosporin	Antibiotic
Baclofen	Lioresal	Muscle relaxant
Beclomethasone	Qvar	Corticosteroid
Benazepril	Lotensin	Antihypertensive—ACE inhibitor
Benzonatate	Tessalon	Antitussive
Brimonidine	Alphagan	Glaucoma agent
Budesonide, formoterol	Symbicort	Corticosteroid and beta agonist
Buproprion	Wellbutrin	Antidepressant
Buspirone	Buspar	Antianxiety
Calcium, cholecalciferol	Vitamin D_3	Calcium supplement
Canagliflozin	Invokana	Antidiabetic—SGLT-2
Carbamazepine	Tegretol	Anticonvulsant
Carbidopa/Levodopa	Sinemet	Anti-Parkinson's agents
Carisoprodol	Soma	Muscle relaxant
Carvedilol	Coreg	Antihypertensive—Beta blocker
Celecoxib	Celebrex	Cyclooxygenase-2 (COX-2) inhibitors
Cephalexin	Keflex	Antibiotic—Cephalosporin
Cetirizine	Zyrtec	Antihistamine
Chlorthalidone	Thalitone	Diuretic—Thiazide
Cholecalciferol, alpha-tocopherol	Drisdol	Calcium supplement
Ciprofloxacin	Cipro	Antibiotic—Fluoroquinolone
Citalopram	Celexa	Antidepressant—Selective serotonin reuptake inhibitor (SSRI)

Generic Name	Brand Name	Drug Class
Clindamycin	Cleocin	Antibiotic
Clobetasol	Temovate	Topical corticosteroid
Clonazepam	Klonopin	Antianxiety—Benzodiazepine
Clonidine	Catapres	Antihypertensive—Alpha agonist
Clopidogrel	Plavix	Antiplatelet
Conjugated estrogens	Premarin	Hormone estrogen
Cyanocobalamin	Vitamin B_{12}	Vitamin
Cyclobenzaprine	Flexeril	Muscle relaxant
Desogestrel, ethinyl estradiol	Apri, Mircette	Oral contraceptive
Dexlansoprazole	Dexilant	Antiulcer agent—Proton pump inhibitor
Dextroamphetamine/ amphetamine	Adderall	Stimulant
Diazepam	Valium	Antianxiety—Benzodiazepine
Diclofenac	Voltaren	Non-steroidal anti-inflammatory drug (NSAID)
Dicyclomine	Bentyl	Antispasmodic
Digoxin	Digitek	Antiarrhythmic
Diltiazem	Cardizem	Antihypertensive—Calcium channel blocker
Divalproex	Depakote	Anticonvulsant
Docusate	Colace	Stool softener
Donepezil	Aricept	Anti-Alzheimer's agent
Dorzolamide/Timolol	Cosopt	Glaucoma agent
Doxazosin	Cardura	Alpha blocker
Doxycycline	Vibramycin	Antibiotic—Tetracycline
Drospirenone, ethinyl estradiol	Yasmin, Yaz	Oral contraceptive
Duloxetine	Cymbalta	Antidepressant—Serotonin and norepinephrine reuptake inhibitor (SNRI)
Enalapril	Vasotec	Antihypertensive—ACE inhibitor
Ergocalciferol	Drisdol	Vitamin D analog

Generic Name	Brand Name	Drug Class
Escitalopram	Lexapro	Antidepressant—Selective serotonin reuptake inhibitor (SSRI)
Esomeprazole	Nexium	Antiulcer agent—Proton pump inhibitor
Estradiol	Climara, Estrace	Hormone, Estrogen
Ethinyl estradiol, norethindrone	Junel, Loestrin	Oral contraceptive
Ethinyl estradiol, norgestimate	Ortho-Tri-Cyclen	Oral contraceptive
Ezetimibe	Zetia	Cholesterol absorption inhibitor
Famotidine	Pepcid	Antiulcer agent—Histamine (H2) antagonists
Fenofibrate	Tricor	Antihyperlipidemic—Fibric acid derivative
Ferrous sulfate	Feosol	Iron supplement
Finasteride	Proscar	Urinary retention agents (drugs used for BPH)
Fluconazole	Diflucan	Antifungal
Fluoxetine	Prozac	Antidepressant—Selective serotonin reuptake inhibitor (SSRI)
Fluticasone	Flonase	Corticosteroid
Fluticasone propionate/ salmeterol	Advair	Corticosteroid and beta agonist
Folic acid	Folvite	Supplement
Furosemide	Lasix	Diuretic—Loop
Gabapentin	Neurontin	Anticonvulsant
Gemfibrozil	Lopid	Fibric acid derivative
Glimepiride	Amaryl	Antidiabetic—Sulfonylurea
Glipizide	Glucotrol	Antidiabetic—Sulfonylurea
Glyburide	Diabeta, Micronase	Antidiabetic—Sulfonylurea
Guanfacine	Intuniv	Nonstimulant cognition enhancer
Hydralazine	Apresoline	Vasodilator
Hydrochlorothiazide	Microzide	Diuretic—Thiazide

Generic Name	Brand Name	Drug Class
Hydrocodone bitartrate	Hysingla	Narcotic analgesic
Hydrocodone with acetaminophen	Norco	Narcotic analgesic
Hydrocortisone	Cortaid, Cortizone	Topical corticosteroid
Hydroxychloroquine	Plaquenil	Antirheumatic agent, antimalarial
Hydroxyzine	Vistaril, Atarax	Antihistamine
Ibuprofen	Motrin	Non-steroidal anti-inflammatory drug (NSAID)
Insulin aspart	NovoLog	Insulin
Insulin detemir	Levemir	Insulin
Insulin glargine	Lantus	Antidiabetic
Insulin human	Regular Insulin	Insulin
Insulin lispro	Humalog	Insulin
Ipratropium	Atrovent	Bronchodilator
Irbesartan	Avapro	Bisphosphonate
Isosorbide mononitrate	Imdur	Nitrates
Lamotrigine	Lamictal	Anticonvulsant
Lansoprazole	Prevacid	Antiulcer agent—Proton pump inhibitor
Latanoprost	Xalatan	Glaucoma agent
Levetiracetam	Keppra	Anticonvulsant
Levocetirizine	Keppra	Anticonvulsant
Levofloxacin	Levaquin	Antibiotic—Fluoroquinolone
Levonorgestrel, ethinyl estradiol	Alesse, Aviane, Tri-Levlen, Seasonique	Oral contraceptive
Levothyroxine	Synthroid, Levoxyl, Levothroid	Thyroid hormone
Linagliptin	Tradjenta	Antidiabetic—DPP-4 inhibitor
Liraglutide	Victoza	Antidiabetic—GLP-1 receptor agonist
Lisdexamfetamine dimesylate	Vyvanse	Stimulant
Lisinopril	Zestril, Prinivil	Antihypertensive—ACE inhibitor

Generic Name	Brand Name	Drug Class
Lisinopril with hydrochlorothiazide	Prinzide, Zestoretic	Diuretic—Combination agent
Loratadine	Claritin	Antihistamine
Lorazepam	Ativan	Antianxiety—Benzodiazepine
Losartan potassium	Cozaar	Antihypertensive—Angiotensin II receptor blocker (ARB)
Losartan with hydrochlorothiazide	Hyzaar	Antihypertensive—Combination agent
Lovastatin	Mevacor	Antihyperlipidemic—HMG-CoA reductase inhibitor
Magnesium	Uro-Mag	Magnesium supplement
Meclizine	Antivert	Antiemetic
Meloxicam	Mobic	Non-steroidal anti-inflammatory drug (NSAID)
Memantine	Namenda	Alzheimer's disease agent
Metformin	Glucophage	Antidiabetic—Biguanide
Metformin with sitagliptin	Janumet	Antidiabetic—Combination agent
Methocarbamol	Robaxin	Muscle relaxant
Methotrexate	Trexall	Antirheumatic agent
Methylcellulose	Citrucel	Laxative
Methylphenidate	Ritalin	Stimulant
Methylprednisolone	Medrol	Corticosteroid
Metoprolol (tartrate)	Lopressor	Antihypertensive—Beta blocker
Metronidazole	Flagyl	Antimicrobial
Mirtazapine	Remeron	Antidepressant
Mometasone	Nasonex	Corticosteroid
Montelukast	Singulair	Leukotriene inhibitor
Morphine	MS Contin, Roxanol	Narcotic analgesic
Mupirocin	Bactroban	Topical antibiotic
Naproxen	Aleve, Naprosyn	Non-steroidal anti-inflammatory drug (NSAID)
Nebivolol	Bystolic	Antihypertensive—Beta blocker

Generic Name	Brand Name	Drug Class
Nifedipine	Procardia XL	Antihypertensive—Calcium channel blocker
Nitrofurantoin	Macrobid	Antibiotic
Nitroglycerin	NitroQuick	Nitrate
Nortriptyline	Pamelor	Antidepressant—Tricyclic
Olmesartan	Benicar	Antihypertensive—Angiotensin II receptor blocker (ARB)
Omega-3-acid ethyl esters	Lovaza	Lipid-regulating agent
Omeprazole	Prilosec	Antiulcer Agent—Proton pump inhibitor
Ondansetron	Zofran	Antiemetic
Oxybutynin	Ditropan	Overactive bladder agent
Oxycodone	Oxycontin	Narcotic analgesic
Pantoprazole	Protonix	Antiulcer Agent—Proton pump inhibitor
Paroxetine	Paxil	Antidepressant—Selective serotonin reuptake inhibitor (SSRI)
Pioglitazone	Actos	Antidiabetic—Glitazones
Polyethylene glycol 3350	GoLYTELY, MiraLax	Laxative
Potassium	Klor-Con, K-Dur	Mineral and electrolyte replacement
Pravastatin	Pravachol	Antihyperlipidemic—HMG-CoA reductase inhibitor
Prednisolone	Orapred	Corticosteroid
Prednisone	Deltasone	Corticosteroid
Pregabalin	Lyrica	Anticonvulsant
Progesterone	Prometrium	Hormone
Promethazine	Phenergan	Antiemetic
Propranolol	Inderal	Antihypertensive—Beta blocker
Quetiapine	Seroquel	Antipsychotic
Ramipril	Altace	Antihypertensive—ACE inhibitor

Generic Name	Brand Name	Drug Class
Ranitidine	Zantac	Antiulcer Agent—Histamine (H2) antagonists
Risperidone	Risperdal	Antipsychotic
Rivaroxaban	Xarelto	Direct oral anticoagulants (DOAC)
Ropinirole	Requip	Anti-Parkinson's agents
Rosuvastatin	Crestor	Antihyperlipidemic—HMG-CoA reductase inhibitor
Sertraline	Zoloft	Antidepressant—Selective serotonin reuptake inhibitor (SSRI)
Simvastatin	Zocor	Antihyperlipidemic—HMG-CoA reductase inhibitor
Sitagliptin	Januvia	Antidiabetic—DPP-4 inhibitor
Solifenacin	Vesicare	Overactive bladder
Spironolactone	Aldactone	Diuretic—Potassium sparing
Sulfamethoxazole with trimethoprim	Bactrim	Antimicrobial—Sulfonamide
Sumatriptan	Imitrex	Serotonin receptor agonists—Triptan
Tamsulosin	Flomax	Alpha blocker
Temazepam	Restoril	Benzodiazepine
Terazosin	Hytrin	Alpha blocker
Testosterone	Depo-Testosterone, AndroGel	Hormone testosterone
Thyroid (desiccated)	Armour Thyroid	Thyroid hormone
Timolol	Timoptic	Ophthalmic beta blocker
Tiotropium	Spiriva	Bronchodilator
Tizanidine	Zanaflex	Muscle relaxant
Topiramate	Topamax	Anticonvulsant
Tramadol	Ultram	Narcotic analgesic
Trazodone	Desyrel	Antidepressant
Triamcinolone	Aristocort, Kenalog, Nasacort	Corticosteroid
Triamterene with hydrochlorothiazide	Maxzide, Dyazide	Diuretic—Combination agent

Generic Name	Brand Name	Drug Class
Valacyclovir	Valtrex	Antiviral
Valsartan	Diovan	Antihypertensive—Angiotensin II receptor blocker (ARB)
Valsartan with hydrochlorothiazide	Diovan HCT	Antihypertensive—Combination agent
Venlafaxine	Effexor	Antidepressant—Serotonin and norepinephrine reuptake inhibitor (SNRI)
Verapamil	Calan, Isoptin	Antihypertensive—Calcium channel blocker
Warfarin	Coumadin	Anticoagulant
Zolpidem	Ambien	Hypnotic

Therapeutic Equivalence

A drug is considered therapeutically equivalent only after demonstrating the same safety and clinical profile when given to patients under the conditions described in the drug labeling. The FDA requires specific criteria be met for a drug to be therapeutically equivalent. This includes the following:

- Approved for safety and effectiveness
- Contains the same active ingredients (pharmaceutical equivalence)
- Uses the same route of administration
- Elicits same effect with same dosage
- Meets the same standards for purity, quality, and strength
- Processed in the body in the same way as the original drug (bioequivalent)
- Manufactured with Good Manufacturing Practices (GMP)

The FDA publishes therapeutic equivalence (and generic equivalence) in the reference *Approved Drug Products with Therapeutic Equivalence Evaluations*, commonly called the Orange Book. The Orange Book identifies equivalence through therapeutic equivalence (TE) codes. These codes are divided into A and B codes. A-codes are considered therapeutically equivalent, while B-codes are not. This enables patients and practitioners to determine generic equivalents for prescribing.

COMMON AND LIFE-THREATENING DRUG INTERACTIONS AND CONTRAINDICATIONS

Drugs can interact with many different substances and diseases, and this can impact the overall effect on a patient. There are several types of interactions that can occur, and these are usually unwanted and can even be harmful.

Drug-Disease Interactions

A drug-disease interaction can occur in a patient if the disease alters the absorption, metabolism, or elimination of a drug. Many drugs are metabolized by the liver and eliminated by the kidneys. If a patient suffers from liver or renal failure, it could impact the way in which a drug is eliminated by the body and result in too high a concentration of drug. Or if a patient is taking a medication to treat one disease, that medication could negatively impact another disease that the patient has. For example, if a patient with urinary incontinence is taking furosemide (Lasix) for blood pressure or congestive heart failure, the patient may have a drug-disease interaction.

Drug-Drug Interactions

When one drug alters the mechanism of another drug, this results in a drug-drug interaction. **Summation** or addition is when the effect of two drugs is the same as the effect each drug would have if taken individually. It is essentially the "sum" of taking the drugs together. If thinking in mathematical terms, this would be equivalent to $1 + 1 = 2$. Alternatively, **synergism** is when the combined effect of two drugs is much larger or longer in duration than the sum of the two. This would be equivalent to $1 + 1 = 5$. An interaction that causes one drug to prolong or increase the effect of another drug is called **potentiation**. This would be equivalent to $1 + 1 = 3$; one of the medications has a higher effect, but the other does not.

If the interaction between two drugs causes one drug to work against the other, this is known as **antagonism**. An example of antagonism is if phenobarbital is taken with warfarin (Coumadin). Phenobarbital actually induces the enzymes that metabolize warfarin. This causes warfarin to be less effective, which can be very dangerous for clot prevention. Antagonistic effects of medications are sometimes used for antidotes or reversal agents.

Drug-Dietary Supplement Interactions

Dietary supplements consist of vitamins, minerals, herbs, or amino acids and are utilized to supplement the diet. These supplements, which are generally all OTC medications, are not tested with the same requirements for effectiveness (they must still prove safety). This also means that the testing is not thorough enough to test interactions with prescription medications and can sometimes lead to dangerous interactions with a medication therapy. It is very important to discuss any supplemental therapy with a prescriber before initiating.

Drug-Laboratory Interactions

Some medications may impact laboratory results and cause false positives or negatives when testing serum levels. Laboratory testing may be conducted through the blood, urine, sputum, or other sample. If a drug causes levels to be misread, there may be a need for additional testing.

Drug-Nutrient Interactions

Drug-nutrient interactions include those found in food or beverages (including alcohol), as well as nutrients in which patients may have a deficiency. Some drugs work better when taken with food, while eating while taking other drugs may impact absorption and reduce effectiveness.

Interaction Type	Example
Drug-Disease	Propranolol and asthma • Beta blockers that are nonselective may cause bronchoconstriction and block the receptors in the airways which respond to asthma medications.
Drug-Drug (Synergism)	Aspirin and warfarin • Both drugs work on the coagulation pathway which may result in bleeding
Drug-Drug (Potentiation)	Sulfamethoxazole and trimethoprim • Sulfamethoxazole potentiates the action of trimethoprim, which increases the antimicrobial action
Drug-Drug (Antagonism)	Ibuprofen and lisinopril • Taking an NSAID with an ACE inhibitor can result in the antagonism of the blood pressure medication, resulting in a reduction in the effect of lowered blood pressure.
Drug-Dietary Supplement	St. John's wort and citalopram • St. John's wort used for OTC depression treatment can modify neurotransmitters in the brain, which can disrupt the action of SSRIs
Drug-Laboratory	Antibiotics and INR (International Normalized Ratio) • If a patient is on antibiotic therapy and taking warfarin, the antibiotic may raise the INR (coagulation test)
Drug-Nutrient (food)	Monoamine Oxidase Inhibitors (MAOIs) and Tyramine • An antidepressant that is an MAOI can cause a significant hypertensive event if a patient eats food with a large quantity of tyramine; this includes aged cheese, smoked meats, hot dogs, and draft beers.
Drug-Nutrient (nutrient)	Antiulcer Agent—H2 receptor antagonist (ranitidine, famotidine) and Vitamin B_{12} • Taking an H2 receptor antagonist such as ranitidine or famotidine may decrease absorption of Vitamin B_{12}.
Drug-Nutrient (beverage)	Atorvastatin and grapefruit juice • Grapefruit juice can increase the absorption of many drugs, which can cause an enhanced effect.

STRENGTHS/DOSE, DOSAGE FORMS, ROUTES OF ADMINISTRATION, SPECIAL HANDLING AND ADMINISTRATION INSTRUCTIONS, AND DURATION OF DRUG THERAPY

Strengths/Dose

The strength of a medication is the amount of active ingredient within a dosage form. This is often expressed in terms of mcg, mg or gram for solids, and mg/mL for liquids. Many drugs are available in more than one strength and dosage form. For example, diphenhydramine is available as 25 mg capsules, 12.5 mg/5 mL oral liquid, and 50 mg/mL IV solution. Drug labels of the most commonly prescribed drugs will include information about specific strengths and dosages, along with any other indications and side effects.

Dosage Forms

A medication may be administered in a variety of dosage forms, depending on the disease treatment and route of administration. A dosage form is the method by which a drug is delivered to its site of action. Each dosage form differs in absorption, distribution, metabolism, and elimination from the body. Dosage forms contain the drug (active ingredient) and generally other inactive ingredients. Some examples of an inactive ingredient include diluents (used to reconstitute or dilute), preservatives (used to slow or prevent the growth of bacteria), and dyes or flavoring agents. While these substances are considered inactive, or inert, and are approved in manufacturing by the FDA, some patients may have a sensitivity to one or more of the inactive ingredients and may even have an allergic reaction.

Dosage forms for medications can generally be broken down into solid, liquid, or semisolid. **Solid** dosage forms include tablets, capsules, powders, lozenges (or troches), and patches. **Liquid** dosage forms include solutions, syrups, elixirs, and suspensions. **Semisolid** dosage forms include ointments, creams, gels, and lotions. Other unique dosage forms include aerosols, inhalants, and suppositories.

Solid Dosage Forms

Tablets are the most popular solid dosage form used for oral administration. Tablets provide a convenient form for patient self-administration, storage, and stability. The onset of action of tablets swallowed is delayed due to first passing through the stomach, then passing into the small intestine for absorption to occur. For this reason, different tablet forms have been developed to allow for faster absorption into the bloodstream. These different tablet types are listed below.

Types of Tablets	Description
Buccal	Placed between gums and cheek and dissolves
Chewable	Designed to be chewed before swallowing
Effervescent	Contains a substance (such as sodium bicarbonate) which reacts with water to give off carbon dioxide (subsequently causing the solution to fizz); must be dissolved before administration
Enteric-Coated	Coated to prevent dissolving in the stomach, intended to bypass and dissolve in the intestine, must not be chewed or crushed
Sublingual	Placed under tongue and dissolves

Capsules contain a gelatin shell which surrounds the active ingredient. It contains a body filled with medication, and a cap that is screwed on tight to the top. Capsules can be opened and sprinkled in food or liquid. The gelatin coating allows for ease in swallowing. Once a capsule is swallowed, the shell must first be digested in the stomach and then the medication can be absorbed in the small intestine. As with tablets, the onset of action is not immediate. The size of capsules ranges from 000 to 5 with the smaller numbers indicating larger-sized capsules.

While most tablets and capsules are designed to release the drug immediately after administration, modified-release dosage forms delay or alter the release of a drug after administration. This may extend the effect of the medication and in turn help with patient adherence. Below are some examples of modified-release dosing.

Drug Abbreviation	Type of Modified Release
CD	Controlled delivery
CR	Controlled release
DR	Delayed release
ER	Extended release
LA	Long acting
SR	Sustained release
TR	Timed release
XL, XR	Extended release

Other solid dosage forms include powders, which are finely ground active and inactive ingredients applied to an external area for treatment or dissolved in a solvent for internal use. Lozenges, also known as troches, are solid dosage forms that contain a flavored base and are designed to dissolve slowly to help expose the drug locally to the mouth and throat. Patches are applied directly to the skin (transdermally) to deliver medication into the bloodstream.

Liquid Dosage Forms

A solution is a liquid dosage form in which the drug is completely dissolved into the solvent. Solutions can be taken orally, injected directly into the body, instilled into the eye or ear, or used as an irrigation or enema. Below is a description of other liquid dosage forms.

Liquid Dosage Form	Description
Irrigation	Used for washing a body cavity (such as the bladder or bowels), a wounded area, or the eyes
Enema	Injected into the rectum for bowel cleansing or to deliver medication
Syrup	A thick liquid that is sweetened with sugar; must be used carefully with diabetic patients
Elixir	A liquid that is sweetened and generally contains alcohol
Suspension	A mixture of particles that do not fully dissolve in liquid; must be shaken well before administration to disperse all particles evenly

Semisolid Dosage Forms

Semisolid dosage forms can mostly be thought of those applied topically to the skin. These include ointments, creams, gels, and lotions. **Ointments** are effective as a skin protectant and have a greasy texture. **Creams** are a semisolid emulsion (mixture of two substances which do not mix) that tend to have a less greasy feel than ointments. **Gels** consist of a jelly-like material with a unique chemical structure that allows liquid particles to be suspended in a solid state. **Lotions** are the least viscous of the semisolid dosage forms and should be applied only to unbroken skin.

Other Unique Dosage Forms

Other dosage forms that fall into an individual, unique group include aerosols, inhalants, and suppositories. An **aerosol** is a suspension of liquid particles that is pressurized to release the particles as a spray. This spray can be inhaled through the mouth as seen with metered dose inhalers (MDI) or through the nose using a mucosal atomizer device (MAD). An MDI delivers a fixed drug quantity into the lungs when inhaled properly. An MAD is attached to a syringe filled with a solution that aerosolizes the medication into a fine mist for nasal inhalation.

Suppositories are unique due to their composition. A suppository is solid at room temperature (or sometimes at refrigerated temperature) but when inserted rectally, the suppository will melt. This allows the medication to be delivered into the body with a quick onset of action (faster than an oral medication).

Routes of Administration

Though many dosage forms are designed for specific routes of administration, many dosage forms can be delivered through multiple routes. Some routes of administration are designed for a local effect only. This means it will act only on the area of the body to which it was applied or instilled. A medication that has a systemic action affects the entire body.

There are three basic routes of administration: **oral**, **parenteral**, and **topical**.

Oral Routes

The oral routes of administration are the most commonly prescribed routes for patients taking prescriptions at home. It is convenient and cost-effective to prescribe medications orally. Though the absorption process does take longer when medications are swallowed, there are other oral routes of administration to utilize when a more rapid action is needed.

To give a medication **sublingually** means to dissolve a tablet under the tongue. By dissolving before swallowing, the medication can be absorbed through the blood vessels in the mouth. **Buccal** route of administration occurs when a table is dissolved between the cheek and gums. This allows the drug to be absorbed through blood vessels in the cheek, producing a more rapid effect. If a buccal or sublingual medication is swallowed, the drug will lose its effectiveness.

Parenteral Routes

Parenteral refers to the administration of a liquid substance (medication or nutrition) into the body through a route that bypasses the intestines. Drugs given parenterally are injected, and therefore not subject to breakdown in the stomach. Though injections may be painful, and while the potential for infection is greater, the absorption of medication is quick and thus a rapid onset will occur. This route is also used in patients who cannot swallow or eat (NPO—nothing by mouth).

Parenteral routes of administration include intravenous (into the vein), intradermal (into the top layer of the skin), intramuscular (into the muscle), subcutaneous (injected under the skin), intra-arterial (into an artery), intra-articular (into a joint), and intrathecal (into the spinal column).

Intravenous (IV) medications are delivered via several different methods. An IV **bolus** is given when a drug must be administered quickly and over a short period. This bolus may be considered a loading dose, which is a large quantity given to a patient to bring the blood concentration of drug to a therapeutic level more rapidly. A bolus is often given using IV push, which is when the medication is "pushed" into the IV line using a syringe.

IV medications may also be administered as an IV piggyback (IVPB) or continuously. An **IVPB** is a small volume infusion (under 250 mL) that is given in addition to a larger volume infusion (it is piggybacked through the main IV). A **continuous infusion** or large volume parenteral (LVP), which is an infusion over 250 mL, provides the patient with a continuous amount of medication over a period of time.

Intradermal (ID) injections are used commonly for testing, such as tuberculosis screening. When an ID is injected, it creates a small wheel, or raised ball of fluid, under the skin.

An **intramuscular (IM) injection** is given directly into the muscle. Most vaccines are administered IM. This injection is given at a 90° angle directly into the skin. IM injections may be painful, and incomplete absorption may result if they are not administered properly.

Subcutaneous injections (SubQ, SC, SQ) are administered directly below the skin but not into the muscle. Patients often inject themselves with medications subcutaneously, such as insulin. A medication given subq should be injected at a 45° angle.

Topical Routes

A medication given topically is applied to the skin or a mucous membrane. Topical routes of administration include transdermal, ophthalmic (into the eye), otic (into the ear), intranasal (into the nose), inhalation, rectally, or vaginally. Topical routes also include application for local treatment using creams, ointments, gels, or lotions.

Transdermal relates to the application of a medication through the skin, and this is typically done via a patch. Fentanyl, nitroglycerin, and nicotine patches are all commonly prescribed for patients. The length of time a patient keeps a patch on (and the point at which they remove it) varies among medications. Transdermal patches deliver medication systemically through the body.

Drugs instilled into the eye use the **ophthalmic** route of administration. This is often abbreviated as OU (both eyes), OD (right eye), and OS (left eye). A medication inserted into the eye can be a solution suspension or ointment.

If a medication is given into the ear, it is done so through the **otic** or aural route of administration. This is abbreviated as AU (both ears), AD (right ear), and AS (left ear). An otic medication may be a solution or suspension. Ophthalmic medications may be used (if necessary) in the ear, but an otic medication may never be used in the eye. This is due to differences in the pH when manufacturing these dosage forms.

It is important to note for both ophthalmic and otic abbreviations that these are considered dangerous and easily confused and should not be used in practice. A pharmacy technician may still encounter these abbreviations on prescriptions, so it is helpful to remember them.

Drugs administered through the **nasal** route are given as a spray through the nostril. This is used often in the form of allergy or saline sprays administered into the nose. Medications inhaled are used to provide a rapid onset of action and deliver medication directly to the lungs. Inhaled medications may be an MDI (aerosol) or through nebules. A **nebulizer** is a machine that helps administer medication into the lungs of patients by conversion of a liquid nebule into a fine mist to be inhaled.

The **rectal** route of administration generally utilizes suppositories and enemas. A suppository is inserted into the rectum for drug delivery into the blood vessels surrounding the rectal area. This leads to a systemic effect. An enema is administered rectally, causing a bowel evacuation in response.

Dosage forms administered **vaginally** include suppositories, tablets, and douches. A douche is a type of irrigation injected vaginally.

A summary of dosage forms that are used for specific routes of administration is below.

Route of Administration	Specific Route Type	Dosage Form Administered
Oral (by mouth)	Oral (swallowed)	Tablet
		Capsule
		Lozenge/Troche
		Solution
		Syrup
		Elixir
		Suspension
	Buccal	Buccal tablet
	Sublingual	Sublingual tablet
Parenteral (bypassing intestines)	IV	Solution
	IM	Solution
		Suspension
	SubQ	Solution
		Suspension
	ID	Solution
	Intra-arterial	Solution
	Intra-articular	Solution
	Intrathecal	Solution (preservative-free)

Route of Administration	Specific Route Type	Dosage Form Administered
Topical (applied to skin or mucous membrane)	Topically	Cream
		Ointment
		Gel
		Lotion
	Transdermally	Patch
	Ophthalmic	Solution
		Suspension
		Ointment
		Gel
	Otic	Solution
		Suspension
	Intranasal	Aerosol
		Solution
	Inhalation	Aerosol
		Nebule
	Rectal	Suppository
		Enema
	Vaginal	Suppository
		Douche
		Tablet

Special Handling and Administration Instructions

Many medications or specific drug classes require special handling when receiving, storing, and compounding or preparing for patient use. Medications deemed hazardous require special garbing of **personal protective equipment (PPE)** when unpacking from wholesaler shipments, counting, compounding, and administering to a patient. Investigational drugs also require special handling to comply with regulatory requirements for experimental drugs used in clinical trials.

Although pharmacy technicians are not generally involved in the medication administration process, it is important to be aware of special administration instructions for specific drugs.

First, the following "five rights" of medication administration should be reviewed:

1. Right drug
2. Right patient
3. Right dose
4. Right time
5. Right route

There is a sixth right (right documentation) that is considered in some institutions. Documenting that a medication was given (or not given) is essential for patient safety. The five rights can be verified through bar-code scanning for medication administration (BCMA). A health care provider can scan a patient's wrist band to confirm correct patient, and then scan the bar code of the medication to confirm right drug, right dose, and right route. Scanning the medication will also alert if it is not the right time.

Some medications have defined requirements for administration, such as administering on an empty stomach or full stomach, taking at bedtime or taking first thing in the morning, if the medication can be crushed or must be swallowed whole, and if there are any restrictions relating to eating or drinking after or before taking. Specific administration instructions for each drug will be included with indications and side effects.

Duration of Drug Therapy

The **duration** is the amount of time a patient will be on drug therapy. For conditions that are **chronic** (i.e., an illness that persists for a long time or reoccurs), the duration may be months, years, or for life. An example of a chronic illness is diabetes. An **acute** illness is one that has a rapid onset, and generally resolves quickly. An example of an acute illness would be a bacterial infection. Duration of drug therapy is also dependent upon patient compliance. **Compliance** is how well a patient follows the medication recommendation from a prescriber. For example, if a patient has an acute infection and is prescribed an antibiotic, but does not finish the recommended course of therapy, the duration of drug therapy may increase if the bacteria becomes resistant to the antibiotic prescribed.

COMMON AND SEVERE MEDICATION SIDE EFFECTS, ADVERSE EFFECTS, AND ALLERGIES

A **side effect** is a secondary effect of a medication, which is outside the anticipated or intended effect, and which occurs within the therapeutic dosage range. Side effects are generally undesirable, although there are few occasions where a drug may be taken for the side effects produced (for example, drowsiness caused by diphenhydramine can be used to promote sleep). Side effects can occur from prescription medications and also OTC drugs. They vary based on route of administration, dosage prescribed, drug class, and patient-specific response.

Patients may notice a side effect if they begin treatment with a new drug, both prescribed and OTC. They may also have side effects if they take more or less than the prescribed dose. Pharmacy technicians can help patients who are experiencing side effects by referring them to the pharmacist for a consultation. The pharmacist can review prescribing and administration as well as discuss ways to reduce the side effects if possible.

Common side effects of medications include the following:

- Drowsiness

- Diarrhea

- Dry mouth

- Constipation

- Headache

- Muscle pain (myalgia)

- Pain at injection site (for drugs administered intravenously, intramuscularly, or subcutaneously)

- Sensitivity to sunlight (photosensitivity)

- Weight gain

Specific side effects of medications will be reviewed with drug indications in the following section.

Severe side effects of medications can also occur. Below are some serious side effects from frequently prescribed medications.

Side Effect	Description	Medications Linked to Side Effect
Stevens-Johnson syndrome	Painful red or purple rash that spreads and blisters	Allopurinol, acetaminophen, ibuprofen, penicillin, anticonvulsants
Reye's syndrome	Serious condition involving swelling in the brain and liver damage	Aspirin (when administered to children)
Tendon rupture	Weakening and rupture of tendons in the shoulder, hand, and heel (Achilles)	Fluoroquinolone antibiotics

Adverse Effects

When a drug causes an adverse event or harm, this is known as an **adverse drug reaction (ADR)**. The American Society of Health-System Pharmacists (ASHP) defines an ADR as an unexpected, unintended, undesired, or excessive response to a drug that results in the following outcomes:

- Requires discontinuing the drug

- Requires changing the drug therapy

- Requires modifying the dose

- Necessitates admission to a hospital

- Prolongs stay in a health care facility

- Necessitates supportive treatment

- Significantly complicates diagnosis

- Negatively affects patient prognosis

- Results in temporary or permanent harm, disability, or death

ADRs can occur at home when a patient is taking a medication, or in a hospital or institutional setting when a drug is administered to a patient. The difference between side effects and adverse reactions is that side effects are generally well-documented and don't require modification of patient treatment.

Some ADRs are considered preventable, including a dosing medication error, an undocumented previous reaction, or a product defect. Nonpreventable ADRs include unforeseen hypersensitivities and genetic reactions. These will vary by patient characteristics, though the older population seems to be impacted the most, especially those who are taking multiple medications concurrently (known as **polypharmacy**). ADRs increase costs to the patient and health care facility if additional medications must be used to treat the reaction, or if the patient must either stay in the hospital longer or be admitted for treatment.

An ADR is often related to the dosage; a patient has an augmented or increased adverse reaction in relation to the dose given. An ADR can also be non-dose related, in which case it is generally **immunologic** or **hypersensitive** (allergic response), or **idiosyncratic** (of unknown cause). Treatment includes discontinuing the drug (if possible), modifying the dosage, and changing drug therapy. Medications may also be used to treat the effects of the ADR. If anaphylaxis (a potentially life-threatening allergic reaction) occurs, epinephrine should be used immediately to treat. If hives or a rash is present, diphenhydramine or a corticosteroid may be used to treat this effect.

Allergies

Although most side effects are well known, allergies are sometimes less predictable due to each person's immune response differing from another. A **drug allergy** occurs when the immune system responds abnormally to a medication. Allergic reactions to medications can be life-threatening, and can also result in hives or rash, anaphylaxis, and swelling of the face and throat. If the airways constrict, wheezing can also occur.

Common triggers of drug allergies are antibiotics, especially penicillins and those containing sulfa. Patients may also experience allergic reactions to the inactive ingredients in a medication, including the dye or preservative used during manufacture. Skin testing can be conducted to determine severity of the allergy. Many times, patients were told they have a penicillin allergy when they were young but are unsure if the allergy is severe enough to warrant non-prescribing. A skin test is a safe way to confirm the allergy and determine whether a different antibiotic is needed.

Treatment for allergies includes avoidance of any product containing the allergen. If anaphylaxis occurs from an allergic reaction, an auto-injection of epinephrine (such as an EpiPen) should be administered immediately.

INDICATIONS OF MEDICATIONS AND DIETARY SUPPLEMENTS

The **indication** of a drug is the purpose or use of that drug in treating a particular disease or condition. For example, the indication for duloxetine (Cymbalta) is depression. Use of a medication for diseases or treatment outside of their FDA-approved indication is considered "off-label" use. This section will give a brief review of the body system for which the drug classes will be described. It will also highlight indications for the top 200 or so medications and special considerations, side effects, dosages, contraindications, and interactions.

NOTE

The following tables are for instructional purposes only. Examples of common generic medications are provided for each drug class, along with the most common dosage and dosage forms (e.g., tablet, capsule, injection, etc). In some cases, all available dosage forms may be listed, but only the most common dosage is provided. Consult the US Food and Drug Administration's website (**www.fda.gov**) for more detailed information.

Cardiovascular System

The cardiovascular system includes the heart and network of blood vessels throughout the body. The **heart** is a muscle that pumps oxygenated blood and nutrients through arteries to be distributed to the cells of the body. **Veins** are blood vessels which carry deoxygenated blood back to the heart. **Capillaries** are tiny blood vessels in which gas exchange (carbon dioxide and oxygen) occurs.

The heart has four valves—two on the top and two on the bottom. The **atria** are the smaller valves on the top, and the **ventricles** are the two larger and more muscular valves on the bottom. The left ventricle pumps blood through the aorta to the rest of the body, so it is the most muscular chamber of the heart. The right ventricle pumps deoxygenated blood to the lungs for oxygenation. The right and left atria are where blood enters—deoxygenated blood in the right and oxygenated blood in the left. Through these atria, blood passes through a valve before flowing into the ventricles. The sound of the valves opening and closing is what makes the "lub-dub" sound when listening to a heartbeat.

When the heart pumps, it pushes against the walls of the blood vessels, creating pressure. **Blood pressure (BP)** has two values: the top value (**systolic pressure**) is when the heart is pumping, and the bottom value (**diastolic pressure**) is the value when the heart is relaxed and filling. Normal BP falls within the range of 120/80 mm Hg.

The heart is composed of an electrical conduction system, which causes an automatic firing of signals to cause the heart to beat. This beat can be recorded through an electrocardiogram (ECG or EKG) which records any abnormalities in a heart rhythm.

Heart disease and disorders are prevalent today and caused by a variety of risk factors. Patient-specific factors could be age, gender, and genetics. Lifestyle-related risk factors include smoking and obesity. The disorders of the cardiovascular system and drug classes for treatment are listed below.

Disorders of the Cardiovascular System

Disorder	Description
Angina	Chest pain resulting from a lack of oxygen supply
Arrhythmia	Abnormal rhythm of the heart
Atrial Fibrillation (AFib)	Irregular, rapid heartbeat
Arteriosclerosis/ Atherosclerosis	Hardening of the arteries due to plaque and cholesterol buildup
Blood Clots	Thrombus (stationary clot) or embolus (moving clot) within a blood vessel
Congestive Heart Failure (CHF)	Weakness in the heart, resulting in its inability to pump sufficiently

Disorder	Description
Hypertension	High blood pressure
Hyperlipidemia	High cholesterol leading to buildup of plaque and cholesterol in the arteries (atherosclerosis), which may lead to hardening of arteries (arteriosclerosis)
Myocardial infarction (MI)	Heart muscle dies after a lack of oxygen and blood supply occurs; also known as a heart attack
Pulmonary Embolism (PE)	Blockage of an artery in the lungs resulting from a downstream clot
Venous Thromboembolism (VTE)	Blood clot in the deep veins (usually legs) that may travel to the lungs, causing a pulmonary embolism

Drug classes indicated for cardiovascular disorders include the following:

- ACE inhibitors
- Alpha agonists
- Alpha blockers
- Angiotensin II receptor antagonists (ARBs)
- Antiarrhythmics
- Anticoagulants
- Antiplatelets
- Beta blockers
- Calcium channel blockers
- Cholesterol absorption inhibitor
- Diuretics
- Fibric acid derivatives
- Lipid-regulating agents
- HMG-CoA reductase inhibitors
- Nitrates
- Vasodilators
- Combination products

DRUG CLASS: ANGIOTENSIN-CONVERTING ENZYME (ACE) INHIBITORS	
Mechanism of Action	Inhibits ACE, which prevents the conversion of angiotensin I to angiotensin II; this results in vasodilation
Contraindications	Liver disease, kidney disorder, pregnancy
Side Effects	Dry cough, hypotension, dizziness
Special Instructions	Must not be taken during pregnancy; fetal mortality can occur
Drug Interactions	Potassium supplements (may cause hyperkalemia), NSAIDs (reduces effect of ACE inhibitor), lithium (may increase blood concentration)

Examples: Angiotensin-Converting Enzyme (ACE) Inhibitors

Generic Name	Dosage	Dosage Form	Indication
Benazepril	5 mg–40 mg PO QD	Tablet	Hypertension
Enalapril	2.5 mg–20 mg PO QD 1.25 mg IV	Tablet Injection	Hypertension, congestive heart failure
Lisinopril	2.5 mg–40 mg PO QD	Tablet, given in one daily dose	Hypertension, CHF (as adjunct)
Ramipril	1.25 mg–10 mg QD/ BID PO	Tablet Capsule	Hypertension, CHF

DRUG CLASS: ALPHA BLOCKERS	
Mechanism of Action	Blocks alpha receptors, which causes vasodilation
Contraindications	Liver impairment
Side Effects	Dizziness, fatigue, headache
Special Instructions	Take first dose at bedtime to avoid dizziness from standing
Drug Interactions	Any other hypertensive agent to avoid significant hypotensive effect

Examples: Alpha Blockers

Generic Name	Dosage	Dosage Form	Indication
Doxazosin	1 mg–8 mg PO QD 4 mg and 8 mg XL PO QD	Tablet Tablet XL (extended release)	Hypertension, benign prostatic hyperplasia
Terazosin	1 mg–5 mg PO QHS	Capsule	Hypertension, benign prostatic hyperplasia

DRUG CLASS: ALPHA AGONISTS	
Mechanism of Action	Stimulates alpha receptors in the brain, which results in lowered blood pressure, heart rate, and vascular resistance
Contraindications	Avoid in patients with recent MI or heart disease, renal failure
Side Effects	Dry mouth, dizziness, headache, fatigue, impotence
Special Instructions	Avoid sudden therapy withdrawal (especially if used together with beta blocker)
Drug Interactions	Tricyclic antidepressants

Example: Alpha Agonists			
Generic Name	Dosage	Dosage Form	Indication
Clonidine	0.1 mg–0.3 mg PO BID	Tablet	Hypertension
	0.1 mg/24hr Q7D–0.3 mg/24hr Q7D	Transdermal patches	

DRUG CLASS: ANGIOTENSIN II RECEPTOR ANTAGONISTS (ARBs)	
Mechanism of Action	Blocks angiotensin II receptors, which prevents vasoconstriction
Contraindications	Pregnancy, patients with low sodium, impaired hepatic or renal function
Side Effects	Headache and dizziness
Special Instructions	If pregnancy is detected, must be discontinued immediately
Drug Interactions	NSAIDs and COX-2 inhibitors

Examples: Angiotensin II Receptor Antagonists (ARBs)			
Generic Name	Dosage	Dosage Form	Indication
Irbesartan	150 mg PO QD and increased to 300 mg PO QD	Tablet	Hypertension, diabetic nephropathy
Losartan	50 mg PO QD, may increase to 100 mg PO QD	Tablet	Hypertension, diabetic nephropathy
Olmesartan	20 mg PO QD, may be increased to 40 mg PO QD	Tablet	Hypertension
Valsartan	80 mg–320 mg PO QD	Tablet	Hypertension, CHF, reduce morbidity following MI

DRUG CLASS: ANTIARRHYTHMICS			
Mechanism of Action	Modifies electrical conduction and force of contraction in heart muscle		
Contraindications	Pregnancy, cardiogenic shock		
Side Effects	Cardiogenic shock, cardiac arrest, CHF, nausea, vomiting, blurred vision		
Special Instructions	Do not take OTC cough, cold, laxatives, or antidiarrheals before consulting physician; amiodarone should be prescribed only by a provider who is familiar with dosing		
Drug Interactions	Warfarin, grapefruit juice, St. John's wort		
Examples: Antiarrhythmics			
Generic Name	**Dosage**	**Dosage Form**	**Indication**
Amiodarone	400 mg PO QD	Tablet	Ventricular fibrillation, unstable tachycardia
	150 mg infused over 10 minutes, then slow infusion of 360 mg over 6 hours	Injection	
Digoxen	0.125 mg–5 mg PO QD	Tablet Capsule	CHF, Atrial fibrillation, atrial flutter
	0.1 mg/mL–0.25 mg/mL	Injection	

DRUG CLASS: ANTICOAGULANTS—WARFARIN			
Mechanism of Action	Inhibits vitamin K, which results in reduced clotting factors		
Contraindications	Pregnancy, surgeries, active bleeding—such as an ulcer		
Side Effects	Unexpected bleeding, alopecia, cramping, nausea, diarrhea		
Special Instructions	Must be taken as prescribed, avoid alcohol, if any new medications are started on warfarin therapy, provider must be notified for dosing modification		
Drug Interactions	Alcohol, antibiotics, vitamin K, steroids		
Example: Anticoagulants—Warfarin			
Generic Name	**Dosage**	**Dosage Form**	**Indication**
Warfarin	2 mg–10 mg PO per day QD or in two divided doses	Tablet	Prophylaxis and treatment of pulmonary embolism

DRUG CLASS: ANTICOAGULANTS—DIRECT ORAL ANTICOAGULANTS (DOAC)	
Mechanism of Action	Inhibits factor Xa in the clotting cascade, resulting in anticoagulation
Contraindications	Active bleeding, mechanical heart valve, liver failure, pregnancy
Side Effects	Bleeding, thrombocytopenia
Special Instructions	Can be taken with or without food and can be crushed
Drug Interactions	NSAID, SSRI, SNRI

Examples: Anticoagulants—Direct Oral Anticoagulants (DOAC)			
Generic Name	**Dosage**	**Dosage Form**	**Indication**
Apixaban	2.5 mg–5 mg PO BID	Tablet	VTE treatment and prophylaxis, non-valvular AFIB
Rivaroxaban	15 mg–20 mg PO QD with meals	Tablet	VTE treatment and prophylaxis, non-valvular AFIB

DRUG CLASS: ANTIPLATELETS	
Mechanism of Action	Binds and modifies platelet receptors, which inhibits platelet aggregation
Contraindications	Active bleeding, liver failure, pregnancy
Side Effects	Upper respiratory infection, chest pain, headache, flu-like symptoms, dizziness, back pain, abdominal pain
Special Instructions	Can be taken with or without meals; alert provider before elective surgery
Drug Interactions	NSAIDs may interfere with metabolism of phenytoin and warfarin

Example: Antiplatelets			
Generic Name	**Dosage**	**Dosage Form**	**Indication**
Clopidogrel	75 mg PO QD	Tablet	Reduction of atherosclerotic events (MI, stroke)

DRUG CLASS: BETA BLOCKERS	
Mechanism of Action	Blocks beta-1 receptor which decreases heart rate and cardiac output
Contraindications	Asthma, bradycardia, diabetes
Side Effects	Dizziness, fatigue, drowsiness, bradycardia, and hypotension
Special Instructions	For patients with diabetes: may mask symptoms of hypoglycemia; avoid abrupt withdrawal
Drug Interactions	Clonidine, NSAIDs, Verapamil

Examples: Beta Blockers			
Generic Name	**Dosage**	**Dosage Form**	**Indication**
Atenolol	50 mg–100 mg PO QD 5 mg/10 mL infusion over 5 minutes	Tablet Injection	Hypertension, acute MI, renal impairment
Carvedilol	12.5 mg PO BID, may increase to 25 mg	Tablet Capsule	Hypertension, CHF, left ventricular dysfunction
Metoprolol	(Succinate) 25 mg–100 mg PO QD (up to 400 mg/day) (Tartrate) 100 mg PO QD (up to 450 mg per day) (Tartrate) 25 mg–50 mg IV Q6H	Tablet Tablet Injection	Hypertension, angina, CHF
Nebivolol	1.25 mg–2.5 mg PO QD up to 10 mg/day	Tablet	Hypertension
Propranolol	80 mg per day up to 640 mg per day in divided doses	Tablet Capsule (sustained release) Injection Oral Solution	Hypertension, arrhythmia, angina, migraines, MI

DRUG CLASS: CALCIUM CHANNEL BLOCKERS			
Mechanism of Action	Inhibits calcium movement of coronary muscles, causing vasodilation and relaxation of muscles		
Contraindications	Symptomatic hypotension, acute coronary syndrome, heart valve defects		
Side Effects	Edema, flushing, headache, fatigue		
Special Instructions	OTC cough and cold medications should not be taken before consulting prescriber		
Drug Interactions	May increase concentration of cimetidine		
Examples: Calcium Channel Blockers			
Generic Name	**Dosage**	**Dosage Form**	**Indication**
Amlodipine	2.5 mg–5 mg PO QD, may increase to 10 mg PO QD	Tablet	Hypertension, angina
Diltiazem	120 mg–240 mg PO QD/BID, may increase to 360 mg/day 10 mg–15 mg/hr IV continuous infusion	Tablet 12hr capsule (SR) 24hr capsule (CD) 24hr tablet (LA) Injection	Hypertension, angina, atrial fibrillation
Nifedipine	30 mg–90 mg PO QD	Capsule Tablet (SR)	Hypertension, angina
Verapamil	80 mg PO Q6–8hr, may increase to total of 480 mg per day in divided doses	Tablet Tablet (SR) Capsule (SR) Capsule (DR) Injection	Hypertension, angina, tachyarrhythmia

DRUG CLASS: CHOLESTEROL ABSORPTION INHIBITORS	
Mechanism of Action	Inhibits the absorption of cholesterol at the small intestine, which decreases amount of cholesterol delivered to the liver
Contraindications	Cannot be used concurrently with a statin by patients with liver disease, pregnant and nursing mothers
Side Effects	Myalgia, abnormality in liver enzymes, rhabdomyolysis
Special Instructions	Do not take within 2 hours of a bile acid sequestrant (Cholestyramine)
Drug Interactions	Gemfibrozil and fenofibrate increase concentration

Example: Cholesterol Absorption Inhibitors

Generic Name	Dosage	Dosage Form	Indication
Ezetimibe	10 mg PO QD	Tablet	Adjunctive therapy with diet for reduction of total cholesterol

DRUG CLASS: DIURETICS	
Mechanism of Action	Acts on different processes depending on diuretic class to increase excretion of sodium, which causes increased excretion of water
Contraindications	Renal dysfunction or electrolyte imbalance
Side Effects	Increased urination, dizziness, thirst, muscle cramps
Special Instructions	Should be taken in the morning to avoid needing to urinate frequently during sleep
Drug Interactions	ACE inhibitors (with potassium-sparing diuretics), digoxin (thiazide and loop diuretics)

Examples: Diuretics

Generic Name	Dosage	Dosage Form	Indication
Chlorthalidone	25 mg–100 mg PO QD	Tablet	Edema associated with CHF, hypertension
Furosemide	20 mg–80 mg PO QD	Tablet Oral solution	Edema associated with CHF, hypertension
	20 mg–50 mg IM/IV over 2 minutes	Injection	
Hydrochlorothiazide	25 mg–100 mg PO QD	Capsule Tablet	Edema associated with CHF, hypertension
Spironolactone	100 mg PO QD, may increase to 200 mg PO QD	Tablet	Edema associated with CHF, hypertension, hypokalemia, hyperaldosteronism

DRUG CLASS: FIBRIC ACID DERIVATIVES	
Mechanism of Action	Lowers total cholesterol, LDL, and triglycerides by increasing elimination of lipids and breakdown of lipids
Contraindications	Hepatic and renal dysfunction; may cause liver toxicity; pregnant and nursing mothers
Side Effects	May cause diarrhea or blurred vision, muscle pain, respiratory disorder
Special Instructions	Do not take if liver, gallbladder, or kidney conditions exist
Drug Interactions	May increase action of warfarin, avoid use with statins

Examples: Fibric Acid Derivatives			
Generic Name	**Dosage**	**Dosage Form**	**Indication**
Fenofibrate	48 mg–145 mg PO QD with meals	Tablet	As adjunctive therapy to diet to reduce cholesterol
Gemfibrozil	600 mg PO BID 30 minutes prior to morning and evening meal	Tablet	Treatment of patients with hyperlipidemia at risk for pancreatitis

DRUG CLASS: LIPID REGULATING AGENTS	
Mechanism of Action	Mechanism of action is not fully understood, but it reduces synthesis of triglycerides
Contraindications	Allergy to fish
Side Effects	Belching, dyspepsia, and taste perversion
Special Instructions	Should be taken with meals
Drug Interactions	May increase bleeding if taken with anticoagulants

Example: Lipid Regulating Agent			
Generic Name	**Dosage**	**Dosage Form**	**Indication**
Omega-3-acid ethyl esters	1 gram PO QID	Capsule	As an adjunct to diet to reduce triglycerides in patients

DRUG CLASS: HMG-CoA REDUCTASE INHIBITORS (STATIN)	
Mechanism of Action	Inhibits HMG-CoA reductase, which is responsible for the synthesis of cholesterol
Contraindications	Pregnancy and nursing, active liver disease, patients who consume large amounts of alcohol
Side Effects	Constipation, muscle pain, dyspepsia
Special Instructions	Avoid overexposure to sunlight (photosensitive); most statins should be taken at bedtime (cholesterol is produced during sleep)
Drug Interactions	Grapefruit juice will increase concentration

Examples: HMG-CoA Reductase Inhibitors (Statin)			
Generic Name	**Dosage**	**Dosage Form**	**Indication**
Atorvastatin	10 mg–80 mg PO QD	Tablet	Hyperlipidemia, reduce risk of MI
Lovastatin	10 mg–40 mg PO QD	Tablet	Hyperlipidemia, to slow progression of coronary atherosclerosis, prevention of coronary artery disease
Pravastatin	10 mg–80 mg PO QHS	Tablet	Hyperlipidemia, reduce risk of MI
Rosuvastatin	5 mg–40 mg PO QD	Tablet	Hyperlipidemia
Simvastatin	5 mg–80 mg PO QD	Tablet	Hyperlipidemia

DRUG CLASS: NITRATES	
Mechanism of Action	Causes relaxation in vascular muscle, which reduces myocardial oxygen demand and lowers pressure
Contraindications	Patients with CHF or hypotension
Side Effects	Headache, nausea, vomiting, flushing of face and neck
Special Instructions	Nitroglycerin should be stored in original glass container and should be administered by dissolving under tongue
Drug Interactions	Hypotensive effect increased with sildenafil (Viagra)

Examples: Nitrates			
Generic Name	Dosage	Dosage Form	Indication
Isosorbide Mononitrate	30 mg–120 mg PO QAM	Tablet	Angina prophylaxis
Nitroglycerin	0.4 mg dissolved under tongue Q5min up to 3 times in 15 minutes	Tablet (sublingual)	Prophylaxis, management, and treatment of angina
	5 mcg/min IV infusion titration	Injection	

DRUG CLASS: VASODILATORS	
Mechanism of Action	Interferes with metabolism of calcium, resulting in relaxation of vascular smooth muscle
Contraindications	Patients with coronary artery disease
Side Effects	Tachycardia, heart palpitations, headache
Special Instructions	Avoid OTC cough and cold agents without consulting prescriber; do not discontinue therapy without first discussing with provider
Drug Interactions	Beta blockers

Example: Vasodilator			
Generic Name	Dosage	Dosage Form	Indication
Hydralazine	25 mg PO QID	Tablet	Hypertension
	20 mg–40 mg IM/IV	Injection	

COMBINATION MEDICATIONS			
Note: In split dosage, the first dosage represents the first medication in the combination, and the second dosage is the second medication. (Example: 2.5 mg/10 mg amlodipine and benazepril = 2.5 mg amlodipine and 10 mg benazepril)			
Examples			
Generic Name	**Dosage**	**Dosage Form**	**Indication**
Amlodipine and Benazepril	2.5 mg/10 mg– 10 mg/40 mg PO QD	Capsule	Hypertension
Lisinopril and Hydrochlorothiazide	10 mg/12.5 mg– 20 mg/25 mg PO QD	Tablet	Hypertension
Losartan and Hydrochlorothiazide	50 mg/12.5 mg– 100 mg/25 mg PO QD	Tablet	Hypertension
Triamterene and Hydrochlorothiazide	37.5 mg/25 mg– 75 mg/50 mg PO BID	Capsule Tablet	Hypertension, edema associated with CHF
Valsartan and Hydrochlorothiazide	80 mg/12.5 mg– 320 mg/25 mg PO QD	Tablet	Hypertension

Respiratory System

The respiratory system is responsible for the inhalation of oxygen and exhalation or removal of carbon dioxide from the body. Oxygen enters the body from either the mouth or nose and passes through the sinuses, which are hollow cavities in the skull. **Sinuses** help filter the air we breathe and regulate the temperature and moisture of the air. Because sinuses are the first contact with outside air, they may become blocked or infected and cause pressure in the skull.

After flowing through the sinuses, air then flows through the **trachea** (also known as the **windpipe**). The trachea branches into two **bronchi**. **Bronchioles** extend from the bronchi, and at the end of the bronchioles are alveoli, also known as **air sacs**. When blood from the heart is pumped to the lungs, gas exchange occurs at the **alveoli**. Carbon dioxide is removed from the blood and exhaled while oxygen from the air we breathe is deposited into the blood.

The **lungs** are organs that contain the bronchi, bronchioles, and alveoli, and are surrounded by a membrane known as **pleura**. The **diaphragm** is located under the lungs, and is the muscle that controls breathing and separates the chest cavity from the abdomen.

Respiratory disorders generally fall into two categories—those caused by infection (either viral or bacterial) and chronic. Many respiratory issues such as coughs and colds are often treated symptomatically with OTC agents.

Disorders of the Respiratory System

Disorder	Description
Asthma	• Inflammation and tightening of the airways • Caused by exercise, allergic reaction, or external allergens • Symptoms include wheezing, coughing, and difficult or labored breathing (dyspnea)
Chronic Obstructive Pulmonary Disease (COPD)	• Chronic obstruction of airflow that interferes with breathing and is not reversible • Comprised of chronic bronchitis (inflammation of lining of the airways) and emphysema (destruction of alveoli caused by smoking, environmental pollution, or infection)
Cough and cold	• Respiratory tract infection most commonly caused by a virus • Characterized by sneezing, itchy throat, coughing (either dry or productive), rhinorrhea (runny nose), and fever • Symptoms are often treated by OTC agents

Drug classes indicated for respiratory disorders include the following:

- Bronchodilators
- Corticosteroids
- Leukotriene inhibitors
- Combination drugs
- Smoking cessation agents
- Antitussives
- Expectorants
- Decongestants
- Antihistamines

DRUG CLASS: BRONCHODILATORS	
Mechanism of Action	Activates beta-2 receptors in lungs, which causes dilation of the bronchioles
Contraindications	Tachycardia, hypertension, coronary artery disease
Side Effects	Nausea, vomiting, nervousness, headache, insomnia, palpitations
Special Instructions	Inhalers must be shaken thoroughly before use
Drug Interactions	MAOIs may increase toxicity; tricyclic antidepressants

Examples: Bronchodilators			
Generic Name	Dosage	Dosage Form	Indication
Albuterol	Two inhalations QID 2.5 mg TID/QID via nebulizer	MDI Inhalation solution (nebule)	Bronchospasm in COPD, maintenance and prevention of bronchospasm
Albuterol and ipratropium	2 puffs QID 3 mL QID via nebulizer	MDI Inhalation solution (nebule)	COPD, bronchospasm
Ipratropium	2 puffs QID, up to 4 puffs 3 mL QID via nebulizer	MDI Inhalation solution (nebule)	COPD, asthma
Tiotropium	18 mcg for use in HandiHaler QD	Capsule	COPD

DRUG CLASS: CORTICOSTEROIDS	
Mechanism of Action	Reduces inflammation, swelling, and mucous production in the airways
Contraindications	Hypersensitivity to milk/lactose (powder in inhalers often contain lactose)
Side Effects	Nasal irritation, congestion, headache, pharyngitis
Special Instructions	Do not exceed prescribed dosage, inhalers should be primed before use
Drug Interactions	Other corticosteroid use

Examples: Corticosteroids			
Generic Name	**Dosage**	**Dosage Form**	**Indication**
Beclometasone	1–4 puffs BID	MDI	Asthma
Fluticasone	44 mcg, 110 mcg, 220 mcg inhalation BID 2 sprays in each nostril QD	MDI Nasal spray	Seasonal rhinitis (nasal spray), asthma (MDI)
Mometasone	2 sprays in each nostril QD	Nasal spray	Prophylaxis and treatment of the nasal spray
Triamcinolone	2 sprays in each nostril QD	Nasal spray	Treatment of seasonal allergic rhinitis

DRUG CLASS: LEUKOTRIENE INHIBITOR	
Mechanism of Action	Blocks the action of leukotriene on receptors in the lungs, which reduces bronchoconstriction and inflammation
Contraindications	Not to be used for asthma attacks or monotherapy for exercise-induced asthma
Side Effects	Headache, cough, influenza
Special Instructions	Should be taken regularly, even when asymptomatic
Drug Interactions	Phenobarbital; may decrease metabolism of paclitaxel and rosiglitazone

Example: Leukotriene Inhibitor			
Generic Name	**Dosage**	**Dosage Form**	**Indication**
Montelukast	4 mg –10 mg PO QPM	Tablet (chewable) Tablet	Prophylaxis and treatment of asthma, relief of symptoms of seasonal allergies, prevention of exercise-induced bronchoconstriction

DRUG CLASS: COMBINATION DRUGS	
Mechanism of Action	Reduces inflammation and swelling and opens the airways
Contraindications	Not to be used for asthma attacks, avoid systemic steroid use
Side Effects	Secondary fungal infections (thrush), upper respiratory infection, pharyngitis
Special Instructions	Rinse mouth after inhalation to avoid fungal infection
Drug Interactions	Beta blockers, MAOIs, tricyclic antidepressants

Examples: Combination Drugs			
Generic Name	**Dosage**	**Dosage Form**	**Indication**
Fluticasone and salmeterol	One inhalation QD Two puffs Q12H	Diskus MDI	Maintenance of asthma, COPD
Budesonide and formoterol	One inhalation Q12H	MDI	Maintenance of asthma, COPD

DRUG CLASS: SMOKING CESSATION	
Mechanism of Action	Mechanisms of action remain unclear
Contraindications	Seizure disorder, MAOIs
Side Effects	Vivid dreams (varenicline), nausea, dizziness, dry mouth, insomnia
Special Instructions	Buproprion dosing is dependent on dosage form, IR is given up to TID, SR is given BID, and XL is given once per day
Drug Interactions	MAOIs, alcohol

Examples: Smoking Cessation			
Generic Name	**Dosage**	**Dosage Form**	**Indication**
Buproprion	100 mg PO TID 200 mg BID 150 mg–300 mg PO QD	Tablet (immediate release) Tablet (SR) Tablet (XL)	Depression, seasonal affective disorder (SAD), management of tobacco cessation
Varenicline (Chantix)	0.5 mg–1 mg PO QD	Tablet	Smoking cessation

The following drug classes are used to treat symptoms of allergies and the common cold. Items that are sold OTC are indicated with an asterisk (*).

DRUG CLASS: ANTIHISTAMINES	
Mechanism of Action	Blocks action of histamine on receptors (histamine causes symptoms of allergies)
Contraindications	Hypertension, glaucoma, diabetes, epilepsy
Side Effects	Dry mouth, drowsiness, dizziness
Special Instructions	Drinking alcohol may worsen side effects
Drug Interactions	Beta blockers and calcium channel blockers

Examples: Antihistamines			
Generic Name	**Dosage**	**Dosage Form**	**Indication**
Cetirizine (Zyrtec)*	10 mg PO QD 10 mg/10 mL PO QD	Tablet Syrup	Allergic rhinitis, urticaria
Diphenhydramine (Benadryl)*	25 mg PO Q4–6H 12.5 mg/5 mL PO Q4–6H 50 mg/1 mL IM or IV up to 400 mg/day Also available in combination cough and cold preparations	Tablet Liquid Injection	Relief of symptoms due to hay fever, allergies, runny nose, sneezing, itchy, watery eyes, and itchy throat, also relieves symptoms of common cold
Fexofenadine (Allegra)*	30 mg–180 mg PO QD	Tablet	Relief of symptoms associated with seasonal allergic rhinitis, urticaria
Hydroxyzine	25 mg–50 mg PO up to QID 10 mg/5 mL PO QID 25 mg/mL–50 mg/mL IV QD/	Capsule Tablet Syrup Injection	Pruritis, contact dermatitis, symptomatic relief of anxiety, sedative for generic anesthesia
Loratadine (Allegra)*	10 mg PO QD	Tablet	Allergic rhinitis, urticaria
Levocetirizine (Xyzal)*	5 mg PO QPM	Tablet	Allergic rhinitis, urticaria

DRUG CLASS: ANTITUSSIVES			
Mechanism of Action	Inhibits cough through anesthetizing receptors in the lungs and reducing cough reflex		
Contraindications	Alcohol should not be used while taking dextromethorphan		
Side Effects	Drowsiness, headache, nausea, dizziness		
Special Instructions	Benzonatate must be swallowed and not chewed or dissolved		
Drug Interactions	Grapefruit juice (dextromethorphan)		
Examples: Antitussives			
Generic Name	**Dosage**	**Dosage Form**	**Indication**
Benzonatate	100 mg–200 mg PO TID PRN	Capsule (Perle)	Relief of cough
Dextromethorphan (Delsym)*	(adults) 10 mL PO BID Also available in combination cough and cold preparations	Liquid	Relief of cough

* sold OTC

DRUG CLASS: DECONGESTANTS	
Mechanism of Action	Stimulates alpha receptors to constrict arteries within the nose and sinuses, causing a decrease in swelling
Contraindications	Hypertension and coronary artery disease
Side Effects	Nervousness, excitability, dizziness, insomnia
Special Instructions	Note when a "D" follows a medication, this means it contains either pseudoephedrine or phenylephrine (indicates a decongestant is added)
Drug Interactions	MAOIs, antihypertensive medications, stimulants

Examples: Decongestants			
Generic Name	**Dosage**	**Dosage Form**	**Indication**
Pseudoephedrine (Sudafed)*	30 mg PO Q4–6H 120 mg PO BID 240 mg PO QD	Tablet Tablet (12hr) Tablet (24hr)	Temporarily relieves runny nose, sneezing, itchy, watery eyes, itching of the nose or throat, and nasal congestion; reduces swelling of nasal passages
Phenylephrine (Sudafed PE)*	10 mg PO Q4–6H	Tablet	Temporarily relieves runny nose, sneezing, itchy, watery eyes, itching of the nose or throat, and nasal congestion; reduces swelling of nasal passages

* sold OTC

DRUG CLASS: EXPECTORANTS	
Mechanism of Action	Increases the output and reduces the thickness of bronchial secretions to promote a productive cough
Contraindications	Hypertension, diabetes, glaucoma
Side Effects	Dizziness, drowsiness, nausea, headache, stomach pain
Special Instructions	If self-medicating, notify provider if cough does not improve after 7 days
Drug Interactions	Alcohol can increase side effects

Example: Expectorant			
Generic Name	**Dosage**	**Dosage Form**	**Indication**
Guaifenesin (Mucinex)*	200 mg–400 mg PO Q4H	Tablet	Helps loosen phlegm and thin bronchial secretions in the bronchial passageway; makes coughs more productive
	600 mg–1200 mg PO BID	Tablet (extended release)	
	100 mg/5 mL– 200 mg/5 mL PO Q4H	Liquid	

* sold OTC

Gastrointestinal (Digestive) System

The gastrointestinal (GI) tract is a tube that starts in the mouth, continues down the esophagus and includes the stomach and small and large intestines, and ends at the anus. The GI system is responsible for the digestion and absorption of food as well as its metabolism and elimination. Food passes through the mouth into the **esophagus** and is then transported (via muscular contractions) into the stomach. Once food is in the stomach, acid is released for breakdown, and then the food moves into the small intestine. The **small intestine** is where nutrient absorption occurs. Once all nutrients have been absorbed, the food passes into the **large intestine** for reabsorption of water back to the body. It then passes through the large intestine to the **rectum**, where it is stored until excretion through the anus. The **gallbladder** assists in digestion by releasing bile, which helps digest fats. In addition, the liver processes the nutrients absorbed from the small intestine.

Many disorders can affect the GI system and some are caused by lifestyle factors, such as poor diet and obesity. Drugs used to treat diarrhea and constipation are generally found as OTC medications.

Disorders of the GI System

Disorder	Description
Gastroesophageal Reflux Disease (GERD)	Also known as heartburn, burning pain in the upper abdomen and chest caused by a reflux of acidic contents of the stomach into the esophagus
Ulcer	A sore formed in the stomach or small intestine caused by hypersecretion of acid
Gastritis	Irritation of the stomach lining that may be linked to medications, alcohol use, and even stress, widespread sores, or ulcers
Crohn's Disease	Inflammatory bowel disease which causes inflammation of the digestive tract, leading abdominal pain, diarrhea, fatigue, weight loss, and malnutrition.
Nausea and Vomiting	Vomiting, also known as emesis, occurs when the stomach or brain is triggered to eject matter from the stomach; nausea is the feeling of sickness, sometimes associated with vertigo or dizziness.
Diarrhea	Loose stools which may be caused by an acute attack from bacterial or viral infection, or chronically by a disorder such as Crohn's Disease
Constipation	Difficulty in emptying the bowels, generally caused by lack of dietary fiber or as a side effect of medication
Flatulence	Gas buildup in the abdominal area

Drug classes indicated for GI disorders include the following:

- Histamine (H2) antagonists
- Proton pump inhibitors
- Monoclonal antibody
- Antiemetics
- Antimotility drugs
- Gut antispasmodics
- Laxatives
- Antiflatulents

DRUG CLASS: H2 ANTAGONISTS	
Mechanism of Action	Inhibits histamine binding at H2 receptors in gastric cells, which suppresses acid secretion
Contraindications	Impaired renal function
Side Effects	Headache, dizziness, constipation, and abdominal pain
Special Instructions	Full course of therapy should be finished; can be taken with food or milk if stomach upset occurs
Drug Interactions	Warfarin

Examples: H2 Antagonists			
Generic Name	**Dosage**	**Dosage Form**	**Indication**
Famotidine	20 mg–40 mg PO BID for 6–12 weeks	Tablet Oral suspension	Short-term treatment of ulcer, treatment of GERD
	10 mg/mL IV Q12H up to 40 mg/day	Injection	
Ranitidine	150 mg PO BID or 300 mg PO QHS	Tablet Syrup	Short-term treatment of ulcer, treatment of GERD, treatment of esophagitis
	50 mg/2 mL IM or IV Q6to8H	Injection	

DRUG CLASS: PROTON PUMP INHIBITORS (PPI)	
Mechanism of Action	Inhibits the proton pump in the gastric cells, which inhibits acid secretion into the stomach
Contraindications	Long-term use has shown increased risk for gastric tumors
Side Effects	Headache, diarrhea or constipation, flatulence
Special Instructions	Take at least 60 minutes prior to eating
Drug Interactions	Increases levels of diazepam, phenytoin, and warfarin

Examples: Proton Pump Inhibitors (PPI)

Generic Name	Dosage	Dosage Form	Indication
Dexlansoprazole	30 mg–60 mg PO QD × 4 weeks	Capsule	Healing of erosive esophagitis, treatment of GERD, relief of heartburn
Esomeprazole	20 mg*–40 mg PO QD × 4–8 weeks 20 mg–40 mg IV over 10 to 30 minutes	Capsule (delayed release) Injection	Healing of erosive esophagitis, treatment of GERD, reduction in occurrence of ulcers, adjunct in *H. pylori* infection
Lansoprazole	15 mg*–30 mg PO QD before meals × 4 weeks 30 mg Infusion	Capsule (delayed release) Tablet (orally disintegrating/SoluTab) Injection	Treatment of gastric ulcers, healing of erosive esophagitis, GERD
Omeprazole	20 mg*–40 mg PO QD × 4–8 weeks	Capsule (sustained release)	Treatment of ulcers, healing of erosive esophagitis, treatment of GERD, adjunct in *H. pylori* infection
Pantoprazole	20 mg–40 mg PO QD × 8 weeks 40 mg/mL Infusion QD × 7–10 days	Tablet (delayed release) Injection	Treatment of erosive esophagitis associated with GERD

* sold OTC

DRUG CLASS: MONOCLONAL ANTIBODY	
Mechanism of Action	Binds to tumor necrosis factor (TNF) and blocks interaction with receptors, this leads to decrease in inflammatory response
Contraindications	Active infections, tuberculosis, autoimmune disease
Side Effects	Headaches, nausea, pain at injection site, infections, and immune reactions
Special Instructions	Must be refrigerated
Drug Interactions	Other biologic drugs such as DMARDs or monoclonal antibodies

Example: Monoclonal Antibody			
Generic Name	**Dosage**	**Dosage Form**	**Indication**
Adalimumab	40 mg/0.8 mL subcutaneously every other week	Injection	Psoriasis, Crohn's Disease

DRUG CLASS: ANTIEMETICS	
Mechanism of Action	Blocks histamine (H1) receptors in the CNS, which blocks the vomiting center in the brain
Contraindications	Asthma, glaucoma, enlargement of prostate
Side Effects	Drowsiness, dry mouth
Special Instructions	Avoid alcohol and use care when operating machinery
Drug Interactions	Increased CNS depression with other CNS depressants

Examples: Antiemetics			
Generic Name	**Dosage**	**Dosage Form**	**Indication**
Meclizine	12.5 mg and 25 mg PO up to 100 mg per day (in divided doses) 25 mg PO up to QID	Tablet Tablet (chewable)	Control of vertigo, motion sickness, not indicated in children under 12
Ondansetron	8 mg PO TID 2 mg/mL slow IV push or infusion over 30 minutes	Tablet Tablet (orally disintegrating) Oral solution Injection	Prevention of nausea and vomiting associated with chemotherapy, nausea and vomiting associated with radiotherapy, postoperative nausea and vomiting
Promethazine	12.5 mg–25 mg Q4–6HR PRN 25 mg, may repeat in 2 hours 25 mg/mL and 50 mg/mL IVPB over 30 minutes	Tablet Syrup Suppositories Injection	Control of motor sickness, control of nausea and vomiting, sedation

DRUG CLASS: ANTIMOTILITY AGENTS	
Mechanism of Action	Binds to receptors to decrease peristalsis (intestinal contraction) and water movement to large intestine
Contraindications	Jaundice, ulcerative colitis
Side Effects	Constipation, drowsiness, nausea, and vomiting
Special Instructions	Discontinue if no response in 48 hours, may cause drowsiness—avoid alcohol, do not take higher dose than prescribed
Drug Interactions	Haloperidol (develop tardive dyskinesia), additive drowsiness effect if taken with CNS depressants

Examples: Antimotility Agents			
Generic Name	**Dosage**	**Dosage Form**	**Indication**
Loperamide (Imodium)*	2 mg PO no more than 16 mg/day	Tablet	Management of diarrhea
Diphenoxylate-atropine (Lomotil)	2.5 mg diphenoxylate/ 0.025 mg atropine PO QID PRN	Tablet Liquid	Management of diarrhea

* sold OTC

DRUG CLASS: GUT ANTISPASMODIC	
Mechanism of Action	Inhibits acetylcholine in smooth muscle which decreases muscle spasm
Contraindications	Urinary tract obstruction, BPH, hepatic and renal disease, CHF and heart disease
Side Effects	Dizziness, headache, nausea, vomiting, dry mouth, difficulty urinating
Special Instructions	Take 30 minutes before meals
Drug Interactions	Haloperidol and phenothiazines

Example: Gut Antispasmodic			
Generic Name	**Dosage**	**Dosage Form**	**Indication**
Dicyclomine	10 mg–20 mg TID/ QID, 30 minutes before meals 20 mg IM QID	Capsule Tablet Syrup Injection	Treatment of irritable bowel syndrome

DRUG CLASS: LAXATIVES (SALINE, STIMULANT, BULK-FORMING, AND BOWEL EVACUANT)	
Mechanism of Action	Promotes evacuation of the bowel through stimulation of fluid or increase in motility
Contraindications	Renal insufficiency, GI obstruction, appendicitis
Side Effects	Diarrhea, nausea and vomiting, electrolyte imbalance
Special Instructions	Should drink plenty of water to avoid dehydration
Drug Interactions	Diphenoxylate/atropine, furosemide

Examples: Laxatives (Saline, Stimulant, Bulk-Forming, and Bowel Evacuant)				
Generic Name	**Dosage**	**Dosage Form**	**Indication**	**Laxative Type**
Bisacodyl (Dulcolax)*	5 mg–15 mg PO QD 10 mg rectally daily	Tablet Suppository	Constipation	Stimulant
Docusate*	50 mg–300 mg PO QD(sodium) 240 mg (calcium) PO QD Insert one enema 1–3 times daily	Tablet Capsule Enema	Constipation	Saline
Lactulose (Enulose)	10 g/15 mL PO QD	Solution	Constipation	Bulk-Forming
Magnesium hydroxide (Milk of Magnesia)*	30–60 mL PO QD	Liquid	Constipation, antacid for indigestion	Saline
Methylcellulose*	500 mg 2 caplets up to 6× per day (no more than 12) 1 scoop QD	Caplet Powder	Constipation and maintenance of regular bowel movements	Bulk-Forming
Polyethylene glycol 3350*	17 grams dissolved in 8 oz	Powder	Constipation and irregular bowel movements	Bowel evacuant

* sold OTC

DRUG CLASS: ANTIFLATULENTS	
Mechanism of Action	Changes the surface tension of air bubbles allowing easier emitting of gas
Contraindications	GI obstruction
Side Effects	Nausea, diarrhea
Special Instructions	Using with alcohol will reduce effect
Drug Interactions	Reduces absorption of tetracycline

Examples: Antiflatulents			
Generic Name	Dosage	Dosage Form	Indication
Aluminum hydroxide-magnexium hydroxide-simethicone (Mylanta)*	10 mL–20 mL QHS and in-between meals	Liquid	Symptoms of gas, indigestion, heartburn, upset stomach
Simethicone (Mylicon) (Gas-X)*	80 mg–125 mg PO TID/QID	Tablet (chewable)	Symptoms of gas
	20 mg PO TID/QID	Liquid	
	0.3 mL–0.6 mL after meals and QHS	Infant drops	
Calcium carbonate-simethicone (Maalox)*	10 mL–20 mL QID PRN	Liquid	Symptoms of gas, acid indigestion, heartburn, upset stomach

* sold OTC

Nervous System

The nervous system is comprised of the **central nervous system (CNS)**, which consists of the brain and spinal cord, and the **peripheral nervous system (PNS)**, which is the surrounding network of nerves. The brain controls both voluntary and involuntary processes in the body. Many of these functions are controlled through the actions of neurotransmitters, which are chemicals released in the brain. Neurotransmitters modulate responses and reactions in the brain, and an imbalance may cause disorders in the nervous system.

Below are some neurotransmitters and the responses they provide. It helps to have an understanding of the function of each neurotransmitter when learning about treatment for neurological disorders.

Neurotransmitter	Function
Acetylcholine (ACH)	Activates muscles in the body; involved in thought, learning, memory and attention
Adrenaline (epinephrine)	Produced during fight or flight response; increases heart rate
Dopamine (DA)	Feelings of pleasure, addiction, and motivation
Endorphins	Released during exercise and creates feeling of euphoria, reducing pain
Gamma-Aminobutyric acid (GABA)	Inhibitory; calming and helps improve focus, low levels contribute to anxiety
Glutamate	Excitatory; involved in learning and memory
Norepinephrine (NE) (Noradrenaline)	Attention and responsive actions in the brain, also causes blood vessels to contract and heart rate to increase
Serotonin (5-HT)	Helps regulate mood, social behavior, sleep, memory, appetite, and digestion

Disorders of the Nervous System

Disorder	Description
Anxiety	A state of uneasiness defined by feelings of apprehension and worry about possible events
Depression	Feelings of pessimism, low self-worth, loss of energy, self-pity, weight loss or gain, and thoughts of death or suicide; often caused by low levels of serotonin or low receptor levels
Bipolar Disorder	Condition characterized by large swings in mood, which include emotional highs (mania) and emotional lows (depression)
Schizophrenia	Neurological disorder characterized by a breakdown in the understanding of reality, emotions, and behavior; false perception of reality causing a withdrawal from relationships, leading to delusional perceptions; thought to be associated with excess dopamine in the brain
Insomnia	Difficulty falling or staying asleep
Epilepsy	Sudden episodes of sensory disturbance, which may include loss of consciousness and convulsions; electrical activity in the brain is abnormal
Parkinson's Disease	Progressive disease which mainly impacts older or elderly patients; characterized by tremors, slow and imprecise movements, rigidity of the muscles and a slow shuffling gait; caused by deficiency of dopamine
Alzheimer's Disease	Progressive deterioration of mental abilities that mainly impacts older adults; leads to dementia and problems with memory, thinking and behavior; low levels of acetylcholine found in patients with Alzheimer's disease
Attention Deficit Hyperactivity Disorder (ADHD)	Symptoms include distractibility, inattention, and poor memory skills; also includes hyperactivity and impulsive behavior
Multiple Sclerosis	Progressive disease caused by damage to the nerve cells in the brain and spinal cord, which leads to impairment of muscle use, numbness, fatigue, and blurred vision
Migraines	Recurring headaches, moderate to severe, that generally last from several hours to a few days; may include nausea and vomiting with sensitivity to light or sound; may be caused by low level of serotonin

Drug classes indicated for nervous system disorders include the following:

- Antianxiety agents
- Benzodiazepines
- Selective serotonin reuptake inhibitors (SSRIs)
- Serotonin and norepinephrine reuptake inhibitors (SNRIs)
- Tricyclic antidepressants (TCAs)
- Monoamine oxidase inhibitors (MAOIs)
- Atypical antidepressants
- Antipsychotics (atypical)
- Hypnotics
- Anti-Parkinson's agents
- Alzheimer's disease agents
- Anticonvulsant (antiepileptic)
- ADHD agents
- Multiple sclerosis agents
- Antimigrainous agents (triptans)

DRUG CLASS: ANTIANXIETY AGENTS	
Mechanism of Action	Exact mechanism of buspirone is unknown
Contraindications	Hepatic and renal failure, may cause tardive dyskinesia (involuntary movements of the face or body) or parkinsonism
Side Effects	Skin rash, tachycardia, headache, fatigue, mood alternation, depression
Special Instructions	May cause drowsiness
Drug Interactions	MAOIs, grapefruit juice

Example: Antianxiety Agent			
Generic Name	**Dosage**	**Dosage Form**	**Indication**
Buspirone	5 mg–30 mg BID, can be given up to four times daily	Tablet	Short-term relief of anxiety

DRUG CLASS: BENZODIAZEPINES	
Mechanism of Action	Enhances the inhibitory effect of GABA, resulting in sedative and anti-anxiety effects
Contraindications	Hepatic impairment
Side Effects	Drowsiness, fatigue
Special Instructions	Avoid alcohol, may be habit forming; do not stop abruptly
Drug Interactions	Other CNS depressants, grapefruit juice

Examples: Benzodiazepines

Generic Name	Dosage	Dosage Form	Indication
Alprazolam	0.25 mg–0.5 mg PO TID, may take up to 4 mg total per day	Tablet (immediate release) Tablet (extended release) Tablet (orally disintegrating) Oral solution	Management of anxiety and panic disorder
Clonazepam	0.5 mg PO TID, maximum daily dosage is 20 mg	Tablet Tablet (orally disintegrating)	Treatment of seizures
Diazepam	2–10 mg PO Q4H PRN 2–10 mg IM or IV Q4H PRN 5 mg–10 mg rectally, max dose is 30 mg	Tablet Injection Rectal gel	Management of anxiety disorders, withdrawal from alcohol, muscle spasm, preoperative apprehension, seizures
Lorazepam	1–10 mg PO QD 2 mg/mL and 4 mg/mL IV push	Tablet Injection	Management of anxiety disorders, insomnia, seizures
Temazepam	7.5 mg–30 mg PO 30 minutes before bedtime	Capsule	Insomnia

DRUG CLASS: SELECTIVE SEROTONIN REUPTAKE INHIBITORS (SSRIs)	
Mechanism of Action	Blocks the reuptake of serotonin, which increases levels of serotonin in the brain
Contraindications	MAOIs (wait 14 days before initiating therapy); antidepressants may increase suicidal thoughts in children and teenagers
Side Effects	Nausea, dry mouth, somnolence, impotence, insomnia
Special Instructions	May impair cognitive and motor performance, avoid alcohol
Drug Interactions	MAOIs, cimetidine, NSAIDs

Examples: Selective Serotonin Reuptake Inhibitors (SSRIs)			
Generic Name	**Dosage**	**Dosage Form**	**Indication**
Citalopram	20 mg PO QD, may increase to 40 mg PO QD	Tablet Solution	Depression
Escitalopram	10 mg PO QD, may increase to 20 mg PO QD	Tablet Solution	Depression
Fluoxetine	10 mg–40 mg PO QD Weekly dose: 90 mg PO QWEEK	Tablet Capsule Capsule (delayed release) Liquid	Depression, obsessive-compulsive disorder, bulimia, panic disorder
Paroxetine	25 mg–62.5 mg PO QD	Tablet Tablet (controlled release) Oral suspension	Depression, obsessive-compulsive disorder, social anxiety disorder, panic disorder
Sertraline	50 mg PO QD, may be increased up to 200 mg/ day	Tablet Oral concentrate	Depression, obsessive-compulsive disorder, social anxiety disorder, panic disorder, premenstrual dysphoric disorder

DRUG CLASS: SEROTONIN AND NOREPINEPHRINE REUPTAKE INHIBITORS (SNRIs)	
Mechanism of Action	Blocks the reuptake of both serotonin and norepinephrine, increasing the levels of both neurotransmitters in the brain
Contraindications	MAOIs (wait 14 days before initiating therapy), glaucoma, hepatic impairment
Side Effects	Nausea, dry mouth, constipation, insomnia, decreased appetite, diarrhea
Special Instructions	Therapeutic effects may take up to 4 weeks to appear
Drug Interactions	MAOIs, antihistamines, NSAIDs

Examples: Serotonin and Norepinephrine Reuptake Inhibitors (SNRIs)			
Generic Name	Dosage	Dosage Form	Indication
Duloxetine	20 mg–60 mg PO QD	Capsule	Depression, neuropathic pain, generalized anxiety disorder
Venlafaxine	75 mg PO QD, may increase to 225 mg/day	Tablet Capsule (extended release) Tablet (extended release)	Depression, generalized anxiety disorder, social anxiety disorder

DRUG CLASS: TRICYCLIC ANTIDEPRESSANTS (TCAs)	
Mechanism of Action	Inhibits reuptake of serotonin and norepinephrine, which increases levels of both neurotransmitters and inhibits action of acetylcholine
Contraindications	MAOIs (wait 14 days before initiating therapy)
Side Effects	Drowsiness, dry mouth, urinary retention, weight gain, tachycardia
Special Instructions	May cause drowsiness, avoid alcohol
Drug Interactions	MAOIs, cimetidine, fluoxetine

Examples: Tricyclic Antidepressants (TCAs)			
Generic Name	Dosage	Dosage Form	Indication
Amitriptyline	10 mg–150 mg PO QHS	Tablet	Depression
Nortriptyline	75 mg–150 mg PO QD/ BID	Capsule Oral solution	Depression

DRUG CLASS: MONOAMINE OXIDASE INHIBITORS (MAOIs)	
Mechanism of Action	Monoamine oxidase is the enzyme which breaks down serotonin and norepinephrine in the brain; MAOIs inhibit this enzyme, which increases levels of neurotransmitters
Contraindications	Liver and kidney impairment, hypertension
Side Effects	Dry mouth, nausea, headache, insomnia
Special Instructions	Must avoid tyramine-containing foods, such as aged cheese, sauerkraut, cured meat; MAOIs should be used in patients who have not responded to therapy
Drug Interactions	Other antidepressants—can create a dangerously high level of serotonin, known as serotonin syndrome

Examples: Monoamine Oxidase Inhibitors (MAOIs)

Generic Name	Dosage	Dosage Form	Indication
Phenelzine (Nardil)	15 mg PO TID	Tablet	Depression (second line therapy)
Selegiline (Eldepryl)	1.25 mg–5 mg PO QD	Capsule	Parkinson's disease, depression

DRUG CLASS: ATYPICAL ANTIDEPRESSANT	
Mechanism of Action	Weak inhibitor of serotonin and norepinephrine reuptake
Contraindications	Pregnancy, patients with recent MI, MAOIs, history of bulimia or anorexia
Side Effects	Insomnia, weight loss, constipation, dry mouth, headache, prolonged erection (trazodone)
Special Instructions	Take in the morning to avoid insomnia (bupropion), take with food (trazodone)
Drug Interactions	Dose-related seizures (bupropion)

Examples: Atypical Antidepressant

Generic Name	Dosage	Dosage Form	Indication
Bupropion	100 mg PO TID 200 mg BID 150 mg–300 mg PO QD	Tablet (immediate release) Tablet (SR) Tablet (XL)	Depression, seasonal affective disorder (SAD), management of tobacco cessation
Mirtazapine	15 mg–45 mg PO QHS	Tablet Tablet (orally disintegrating)	Depression
Trazodone	50 mg–300 mg PO max daily dose is 400 mg	Tablet	Depression

DRUG CLASS: ANTIPSYCHOTICS	
Mechanism of Action	Exact mechanism is unknown, thought to act on dopamine receptors as an antagonist
Contraindications	History of seizures, cardiovascular disease, dementia-related psychosis
Side Effects	Headache, weight gain, insomnia, tardive dyskinesia
Special Instructions	Avoid alcohol, may cause fainting (risperidone)
Drug Interactions	Carbamazepine, fluoxetine, paroxetine

Examples: Antipsychotics

Generic Name	Dosage	Dosage Form	Indication
Aripiprazole	10 mg–15 mg PO QD	Tablet Tablet (orally disintegrating) Oral solution	Schizophrenia, bipolar disorder
Quetiapine	300 mg–400 mg PO QD in 2 or 3 divided doses	Tablet Tablet (extended release)	Schizophrenia, bipolar disorder
Risperidone	1 mg PO BID, maximum daily dose is 16 mg	Tablet Tablet (orally disintegrating) Oral solution	Schizophrenia, bipolar disorder, irritability associated with autism
	25 mg–50 mg IM Q2WEEKS	Injection	

DRUG CLASS: HYPNOTICS	
Mechanism of Action	Interacts with GABA receptors and causes sedation
Contraindications	Depression, renal impairment
Side Effects	Headache, drowsiness, nausea
Special Instructions	May cause sleep driving, or other activities the patient does not recall happening
Drug Interactions	Other CNS depressants

Example: Hypnotics

Generic Name	Dosage	Dosage Form	Indication
Zolpidem	5–10 mg PO QHS	Tablet	Insomnia
	6.25 mg–12.5 mg PO QHS	Tablet (controlled release)	

DRUG CLASS: ANTI-PARKINSON'S AGENTS	
Mechanism of Action	Increases levels of dopamine in the brain
Contraindications	Smoking increases concentration in the blood
Side Effects	Nausea, dizziness, somnolence, syncope, fatigue, involuntary movements
Special Instructions	May cause abrupt onset of sleep; avoid driving or operating machinery
Drug Interactions	Omeprazole, ciprofloxacin, MAOI can cause hypertensive crisis

Examples: Anti-Parkinson's Agents			
Generic Name	Dosage	Dosage Form	Indication
Carbidopa-levodopa (dosage is indicated with carbidopa as the first dosage and levodopa second)	10 mg/100 mg PO TID– 25 mg/250 mg PO TID 25 mg/100 mg PO BID– 50 mg/200 mg PO BID	Tablet Tablet (controlled release)	Parkinson's disease
Ropinirole	0.25 mg–5 mg PO TID 2 mg–8 mg PO QD	Tablet Tablet (extended release)	Parkinson's disease, restless leg syndrome

DRUG CLASS: ALZHEIMER'S DISEASE AGENTS	
Mechanism of Action	Increases acetylcholine in the brain—Alzheimer's is characterized by a deficiency in acetylcholine (Donepezil)
Contraindications	May increase gastric acid secretion (use caution in patients with GI bleed)
Side Effects	Nausea, diarrhea, insomnia, anorexia
Special Instructions	Take before bed
Drug Interactions	Phenytoin, carbamazepine; phenobarbital and dexamethasone increase metabolism

Examples: Alzheimer's Disease Agents			
Generic Name	Dosage	Dosage Form	Indication
Donepezil	5 mg–10 mg PO QHS	Tablet Tablet (orally disintegrating) Oral solution	Mild, moderate, and severe dementia caused by Alzheimer's disease
Memantine	20 mg PO QD	Tablet Oral solution	Moderate, and severe dementia caused by Alzheimer's disease

DRUG CLASS: ANTICONVULSANT (ANTIEPILEPTIC)	
Mechanism of Action	Either decrease excitatory (glutamate) neurotransmission or increase inhibitory (GABA) neurotransmission
Contraindications	MAOIs (wait 14 days before initiating therapy)
Side Effects	Dizziness, unsteadiness, life-threatening rashes (lamotrigine)
Special Instructions	Drink a full glass of water after administration (carbamazepine)
Drug Interactions	Warfarin, grapefruit juice, antacids (gabapentin)

Examples: Anticonvulsant (Antiepileptic)			
Generic Name	Dosage	Dosage Form	Indication
Carbamazepine	800 mg–1200 mg per day in 3 or 4 divided doses	Tablet Tablet (chewable) Tablet (extended release) Capsule (extended release) Suspension	Seizure disorder
Divalproex	250 mg PO TID	Tablet (enteric-coated) Tablet (extended release) Sprinkle capsules	Seizure disorder, bipolar disorder, prophylaxis of migraines
Gabapentin	300 mg–600 mg PO TID	Capsule Tablet Oral solution	Adjunctive therapy for seizure disorder, postherpetic neuralgia
Lamotrigine	25 mg–200 mg PO QD	Tablet (chewable) Tablet (orally disintegrating) Tablet (extended release)	Adjunctive therapy for seizure disorder, bipolar disorder
Levetiracetam	500 mg PO BID	Tablet (immediate release) Tablet (extended release) Oral solution	Adjunctive therapy for seizure disorder
Pregabalin	25 mg–225 mg PO TID	Capsule	Adjunctive therapy for seizure disorder, fibromyalgia, neuropathic pain
Topiramate	25 mg–200 mg PO QHS	Tablet	Adjunctive therapy for seizure disorder, prophylaxis for migraines

DRUG CLASS: ADHD AGENTS	
Mechanism of Action	Stimulants, which increase levels of norepinephrine and dopamine, speeding up brain activity
Contraindications	Hyperthyroidism, hypertension, patients with history of drug abuse
Side Effects	Restlessness, dizziness, insomnia, anorexia
Special Instructions	May be habit forming
Drug Interactions	MAOIs may cause hypertensive crisis

Examples: ADHD Agents			
Generic Name	**Dosage**	**Dosage Form**	**Indication**
Dextroamphetamine and amphetamine	20 mg PO QD	Tablet Capsule	Narcolepsy, ADHD
Guanfacine	1 mg PO QD—taken at the same time every day	Tablet Tablet (extended release)	ADHD
Lisdexamfetamine	30 mg PO QAM, may increase up to 70 mg/day	Capsule	ADHD in children 6 years and older
Methylphenidate	18–54 mg PO QD	Tablet Tablet (sustained release) Capsule (controlled release) Tablet (chewable) Solution	ADHD in children 6 years and older, narcolepsy

DRUG CLASS: AGENTS FOR MULTIPLE SCLEROSIS (MS)	
Mechanism of Action	Agonist of GABA which increases inhibitory action
Contraindications	Impaired renal function, epilepsy, history of stroke
Side Effects	Drowsiness, dizziness, headache, insomnia, abnormal liver function tests
Special Instructions	Avoid alcohol
Drug Interactions	Other CNS depressants, oral contraceptives (tizanidine)

Examples: Agents for Multiple Sclerosis (MS)			
Generic Name	**Dosage**	**Dosage Form**	**Indication**
Baclofen	10 mg–20 mg PO TID/QID	Tablet	Spasticity resulting from MS
Tizanidine	4 mg PO Q6–8HR with maximum of 3 doses in 24 hours	Tablet	Spasticity resulting from MS

DRUG CLASS: ANTIMIGRAINOUS AGENTS—TRIPTANS	
Mechanism of Action	Selective agonist of serotonin receptors
Contraindications	Cannot be administered intravenously
Side Effects	Abnormal tingling, warmth, or burning, flushing
Special Instructions	Administer as soon as symptoms of migraine appear; does not prevent migraines
Drug Interactions	MAOIs

Example: Antimigrainous Agent—Triptans			
Generic Name	Dosage	Dosage Form	Indication
Sumatriptan	25 mg–100 mg PO at onset	Tablet	Treatment of migraines
	4 mg and 6 mg syringes at onset	Injection	
	5 mg and 20 mg nasal spray at onset	Nasal spray	

Urinary System

The urinary or renal system functions to maintain the proper balance of water and electrolytes throughout the body, including the fluid in plasma and tissues. This results in excretion and formation of urine or reabsorption of water and electrolytes back into the bloodstream.

The **kidneys** contain the main working unit of the urinary system, known as the **nephron**. The nephrons produce the urine through filtration, reabsorption, and secretion. These processes help maintain blood pressure and keep the blood clean of waste, while reabsorbing what the body needs and excreting what is not needed. Within the **glomerulus** is the **renal tubule**, which houses the proximal convoluted tubule, loop of Henle, distal convoluted tubule, and connecting tubule. Each portion of the renal tubule excretes or reabsorbs specific substances. Medications may act on specific portions to impact reabsorption or secretion of certain nutrients or electrolytes.

From the renal tubule, the **urine** flows into the collecting duct and then into the **ureters**. The ureters are tubes connecting the kidneys to the bladder. The **bladder** is the storage container for urine until the body is ready to void or excrete it from the body. From the bladder, urine travels through the urethra to out of the body. The **urethra** in men is much longer than women, though the remainder of the urinary system in men and women is the same. The shortened urethra in women leads to a higher incident of urinary tract infections due to the short proximity from the urethra to the bladder.

Disorders of the Urinary System

Disorder	Description
Benign Prostatic Hyperplasia (BPH)	Abnormal enlargement of the prostate gland in men; obstructs urine outflow
Cystitis	Urinary tract infection (UTI); symptoms include pain when urinating, blood in the urine, and a constant urge to urinate
Gout	A form of arthritis causing tenderness in the joints due to a large amount of uric acid; uric acid is usually excreted in the urine
Overactive Bladder	Defined as voiding urine 8 or more times in a 24-hour period or waking more than 2 times during the night to urinate
Hypertension	High blood pressure; often treated with diuretics

Drug Classes indicated for urinary system disorders include the following:

- Alpha blockers
- Urinary retention agents (drugs used for BPH)
- Antimicrobial agents
- Antigout agents
- Overactive bladder agents
- Diuretics
  - Thiazide diuretic
  - Loop diuretic
  - Potassium-sparing diuretic
  - Combination drugs

DRUG CLASS: ALPHA BLOCKERS			
Mechanism of Action	Blocks alpha receptors, which causes vasodilation		
Contraindications	Liver impairment		
Side Effects	Dizziness, fatigue, headache		
Special Instructions	Take first dose at bedtime to avoid dizziness from standing		
Drug Interactions	Any other hypertensive agent to avoid significant hypotensive effect		
Examples: Alpha Blockers			
Generic Name	**Dosage**	**Dosage Form**	**Indication**
Doxazosin	1 mg–8 mg PO QD 4 mg and 8 mg XL PO QD	Tablet Tablet (XL)	Hypertension, BPH
Tamsulosin	0.4 mg PO QD following same meal daily	Capsule	BPH
Terazosin	1 mg–10 mg PO QHS	Capsule	Hypertension, BPH

DRUG CLASS: URINARY RETENTION AGENTS (DRUGS USED FOR BPH)			
Mechanism of Action	Inhibits enzyme which normally metabolizes testosterone		
Contraindications	Women and children		
Side Effects	Impotence, decreased libido		
Special Instructions	Women who plan to become pregnant should not handle or be exposed to semen from man who is taking		
Drug Interactions	Decreases theophylline levels		
Example: Urinary Retention Agent (Drugs used for BPH)			
Generic Name	**Dosage**	**Dosage Form**	**Indication**
Finasteride	5 mg PO QD	Tablet	BPH

DRUG CLASS: ANTIMICROBIAL AGENTS	
Mechanism of Action	Inhibits growth or kills bacteria
Contraindications	Sulfa allergies, penicillin allergies, hepatic or renal impairment
Side Effects	Photosensitivity, Stevens-Johnson syndrome (Bactrim)
Special Instructions	Avoid prolonged exposure to sunlight
Drug Interactions	Warfarin

Examples: Antimicrobial Agents			
Generic Name	**Dosage**	**Dosage Form**	**Indication**
Amoxicillin	250 mg–500 mg PO Q8H or 500 mg–875 mg Q12H	Tablet (chewable) Tablet Capsule Oral suspension	UTI, infections due to *E.coli* and gram-positive organisms, gonorrhea
Amoxicillin and clavulanate	250 mg–500 mg PO Q8H or Q12H	Tablet (chewable) Tablet (extended release) Oral suspension	Recurrent otitis media, UTI, bacterial sinusitis
Cephalexin	250 mg–1000 mg PO Q6H	Capsule Tablet Oral suspension	UTI, infections due to *E.coli*
Ciprofloxacin	250 mg–500 mg PO Q12H or 500 mg–1000 mg PO QD	Tablet Tablet (extended release) Oral suspension Injection	Infection diarrhea, UTI, gonorrhea, cystitis, bone/joint infections
Levofloxacin	250 mg–750 mg PO Q24H	Tablet Oral Solution Injection	Community acquired pneumonia, UTI, sinusitis, anthrax
Nitrofurantoin	100 mg PO Q12H × 7 days	Capsule	UTI
Sulfamethoxazole and trimethoprim	800 mg sulfamethoxazole / 160 mg trimethoprim Q12H × 10–14 days	Tablet (regular strength) Tablet (double strength) Oral suspension Injection	UTI, otitis media

Drug Class: Antigout Agents	
Mechanism of Action	Inhibits the enzyme that creates uric acid
Contraindications	Renal or hepatic impairment
Side Effects	Drowsiness, diarrhea, nausea and vomiting
Special Instructions	High fluid intake is important to prevent kidney stone formation
Drug Interactions	May increase rash when used with ampicillin

Example: Antigout Agent			
Generic Name	**Dosage**	**Dosage Form**	**Indication**
Allopurinol	200 mg–300 mg per day for mild 400 mg–600 mg per day for severe	Tablet Injection	Treatment of gout

DRUG CLASS: OVERACTIVE BLADDER AGENTS	
Mechanism of Action	Blocks the receptors involved in contraction of urinary muscles
Contraindications	Patients with urinary or gastric retention, bladder obstruction
Side Effects	Dry mouth, UTI, constipation
Special Instructions	Avoid prolonged exposure to hot weather, may cause dizziness
Drug Interactions	Clarithromycin (solifenacin), haloperidol (oxybutynin)

Examples: Overactive Bladder Agents			
Generic Name	**Dosage**	**Dosage Form**	**Indication**
Oxybutynin	5 mg PO QD, may increase to maximum of 30 mg per day	Tablet Tablet (extended release) Syrup	Treatment of overactive bladder
Solifenacin	5 mg PO QD, may be increased to 10 mg	Tablet	Treatment of overactive bladder

DRUG CLASS: DIURETICS—THIAZIDE	
Mechanism of Action	Inhibits reabsorption of sodium and chloride at distal renal tubule
Contraindications	Sulfa allergies, patients with gout, impaired renal or hepatic functions, diabetes
Side Effects	Dry mouth, muscle cramps, nausea and vomiting, anemia, photosensitivity
Special Instructions	Take early in AM, avoid excessive exposure to sunlight
Drug Interactions	Lithium; may cause hyperglycemia

Examples: Diuretics—Thiazide			
Generic Name	**Dosage**	**Dosage Form**	**Indication**
Chlorthalidone	25 mg–100 mg PO QD	Tablet	Adjunctive therapy in edema associated with CHF or renal dysfunction, hypertension
Hydrochlorothiazide	25 mg–100 mg PO QD	Tablet	Adjunctive therapy in edema associated with CHF or renal dysfunction, hypertension

DRUG CLASS: DIURETICS—LOOP	
Mechanism of Action	Inhibits sodium and chloride reabsorption in the loop of Henle
Contraindications	Severe electrolyte depletion
Side Effects	Impaired hearing, hypotension, muscle cramps, hyponatremia, hypochloremia
Special Instructions	Take early in AM
Drug Interactions	Aminoglycosides and cisplatin increase auditory toxicity

Examples: Diuretics—Loop			
Generic Name	**Dosage**	**Dosage Form**	**Indication**
Bumetanide	0.5 mg–2 mg PO QD, max of 10 mg/day	Tablet	Treatment of edema associated with CHF or renal dysfunction
	0.5 mg–1 mg IM or IV push given over 1–2 minutes	Injection	
Furosemide	20 mg–80 mg PO QD, may increase 20–40 mg up to 600 mg	Tablet Oral solution	Treatment of edema associated with CHF or renal dysfunction, hypertension, pulmonary edema
	40 mg IV Push over 1–2 minutes	Injection	

DRUG CLASS: DIURETICS—POTASSIUM-SPARING	
Mechanism of Action	Blocks the effect of aldosterone, which results in the secretion of sodium
Contraindications	Hepatic failure, fluid and electrolyte disturbances
Side Effects	Dry mouth, muscle cramps, amenorrhea, headache, weakness
Special Instructions	Take early in a.m.
Drug Interactions	Should not be used with ACE inhibitors, as the potassium-sparing effects of these can lead to hyperkalemia

Examples: Diuretics—Potassium-sparing			
Generic Name	**Dosage**	**Dosage Form**	**Indication**
Spironolactone	100 mg PO QD, may increase to 200 mg PO QD	Tablet	Edema associated with CHF, hypertension, hypokalemia, hyperaldosteronism

Examples: Combination Diuretics			
Note: The following are combination medications, which include an antihypertensive agent with a diuretic for an additive effect on blood pressure.			
Generic Name	**Dosage**	**Dosage Form**	**Indication**
Lisinopril and Hydrochlorothiazide	10 mg lisinopril/12.5 mg hydrochlorothiazide to 20 mg lisinopril/25 mg hydrochlorothiazide PO QD	Tablet	Hypertension
Losartan and Hydrochlorothiazide	50 mg losartan/12.5 mg hydrochlorothiazide to 100 mg losartan /25 mg hydrochlorothiazide PO QD	Tablet	Hypertension
Triamterene and Hydrochlorothiazide	37.5 mg triamterene/ 25 mg hydrochlorothiazide to 75 mg triamterene/50 mg hydrochlorothiazide PO QD/BID	Tablet Capsule	Hypertension, Adjunctive therapy in edema associated with CHF or renal dysfunction
Hydrochlorothiazide and Valsartan	80 mg valsartan/ 12.5 mg hydrochlorothiazide to 320 mg valsartan /25 mg hydrochlorothiazide PO QD	Tablet	Hypertension

Endocrine System

The endocrine system is a system of glands and other structures that produce or secrete hormones. These hormones keep the body in **homeostasis**, or physiological equilibrium. The **endocrine system** consists of the following glands and organs: pituitary gland, thyroid gland, hypothalamus, pineal gland parathyroid gland, adrenal gland, thymus gland, ovaries, testes, and pancreas.

The **pituitary gland** produces nine hormones that impact various parts of the body. The **thyroid gland** secretes three hormones that are important for metabolism. The **hypothalamus** helps regulate the autonomic nervous system and links the brain with the endocrine system through the pituitary gland. The **pineal gland** is important for sleep cycles. The **parathyroid gland** helps maintain appropriate levels of calcium in the body. The **adrenal glands** secrete glucocorticoids and epinephrine and norepinephrine. The **thymus gland** plays an important role in immunity. The **ovaries and testes** are involved in reproduction and hormone release for female and male sex characteristics. The **pancreas** releases insulin and glucagon to regulate sugar in the blood.

Below are functions of glands and organs of the endocrine system.

Gland	Secretes or Produces	Site of Action	Function
Pituitary	Antidiuretic hormone (ADH) also known as vasopressin	Kidneys	Balances amount of water in blood
	Oxytocin (OT)	Uterine muscle and mammary glands	Stimulates lactation, as well as contractions during childbirth
	Prolactin	Mammary glands	Induces lactation
	Melanocyte-stimulating hormone	Skin	Stimulates release of melanin in skin
	Follicle-stimulating hormone (FSH)	Ovary and testes	Stimulates growth of follicles in ovaries, and testicular growth in men
	Luteinizing hormone (LH)	Ovary and testes	Causes ovulation in women, and works in conjunction with FSH in men
	Thyroid-stimulating hormone (TSH)	Thyroid	Induces the thyroid to produce thyroid hormones
	Adrenocorticotropic hormone (ACTH)	Adrenal gland	Regulates amount of cortisol released from adrenal gland
	Growth hormone	Bones	Causes growth in children and regulates muscle and bone composition in adults

Gland	Secretes or Produces	Site of Action	Function
Thyroid	Triiodothyronine (T3)	Bloodstream	Regulates (along with T4) temperature, metabolism, and heart rate
	Thyroxine (T4)	Bloodstream	Regulates (along with T3) temperature, metabolism, and heart rate
	Calcitonin	Bloodstream	Reduces calcium levels in the blood
Pineal	Melatonin	Bloodstream	Regulation of sleep cycle
Parathyroid	Parathyroid Hormone (PTH)	Bloodstream	Increases calcium levels in the blood
Adrenal	Epinephrine (Adrenaline)	Bloodstream	Increases heart rate in response to stress
	Norepinephrine (Noradrenaline)	Bloodstream	Increases heart rate in response to stress
	Cortisol	Bloodstream	Steroid hormone released in response to stress or low glucose
	Aldosterone	Bloodstream	Steroid hormone which increases sodium reabsorption in kidneys
Thymus	Thymosin	Bloodstream	T-cell development and production
Ovaries	Estrogen	Bloodstream	T-cell development and production
	Progesterone	Bloodstream	Regulates endometrial lining
Testes	Testosterone	Bloodstream	Male sex characteristic development
Pancreas	Insulin	Bloodstream	Decreases blood sugar by converting into glycogen for storage
	Glucagon	Bloodstream	Causes liver to convert stored glycogen into insulin, increasing blood sugar

Disorders of the Endocrine System

Disorder	Endocrine Gland Affected	Description
Hypothyroidism	Thyroid	Production of thyroid hormone is below normal
Hyperthyroidism	Thyroid	Excessive level of thyroid hormone
Addison's disease	Adrenal	Deficiency in steroid hormones, which causes weight loss, low blood pressure, and excess potassium
Diabetes Type I	Pancreas	Insulin-dependent diabetes—the body does not produce insulin
Diabetes Type II	Pancreas	Insulin resistance in the pancreas—the body does not respond to insulin, so glucose is not absorbed
Osteoporosis	Ovaries and Parathyroid	Bone resorption exceeds new bone production, which causes weakening of bones and less density; occurs as a result of deficiency in estrogen, calcium, and vitamin D
Hypogonadism	Testes	Deficient production and secretion of testosterone
Hormone Replacement	Ovaries	Used to treat the symptoms of menopause
Menstrual Dysfunction	Ovaries	Includes amenorrhea (absence of menstruation), dysmenorrhea (difficult or painful menstruation), endometriosis (endometrium grows outside of uterus), and abnormal bleeding

Drug classes indicated for endocrine system disorders include the following:

- Thyroid hormone
- Corticosteroids
- Hypoglycemic agents
- Insulin
- Bisphosphonates
- Androgens
- Oral contraceptives
- Hormone replacement
- Progestin hormones

DRUG CLASS: THYROID HORMONE	
Mechanism of Action	Synthetic form of T4 which is converted to T3
Contraindications	Adrenal cortical insufficiency, cardiovascular disorders, diabetes, anticoagulants
Side Effects	Hypoglycemia, fluid loss, tachycardia
Special Instructions	May cause hair loss in children; do not discontinue therapy without consult
Drug Interactions	Warfarin may decrease effect of digoxin

Examples: Thyroid Hormone			
Generic Name	**Dosage**	**Dosage Form**	**Indication**
Levothyroxine	25 mcg–300 mcg PO QD 100 mcg–300 mcg IV	Tablet Injection	Replacement therapy for absent thyroid function
Thyroid (desiccated)	60 mg–180 mg PO QD	Tablet	Hypothyroidism, treatment or prevention of goiter

DRUG CLASS: CORTICOSTEROIDS	
Mechanism of Action	Suppresses the reactions of the immune system for an anti-inflammatory action
Contraindications	Systemic fungal infection, hypothyroidism, renal impairment, patients on immunosuppressant agents
Side Effects	Blurred vision, upset stomach, myopathy
Special Instructions	May take with food if GI upset occurs, increased susceptibility for infection
Drug Interactions	Long-term use may diminish response to vaccines

Examples: Corticosteroids			
Generic Name	**Dosage**	**Dosage Form**	**Indication**
Hydrocortisone	15 mg–240 mg IM or Infusion Q12H	Injection Cream Ointment	Allergic reaction
Methylprednisolone	4 mg–48 mg PO QD Dosepak: 21 tablet pack with incremental increase	Tablet Dosepak Injection	Allergic and inflammatory disease
Prednisone	5 mg–60 mg PO QD	Tablet Oral Solution	Allergic and inflammatory disease
Prednisolone	5 mg–60 mg PO QD	Oral solution	Allergic and inflammatory disease
Triamcinolone	40–80 mg IM once	Injection	Allergic reaction

DRUG CLASS: HYPOGLYCEMIC AGENTS	
Mechanism of Action	Stimulates insulin release from beta cells in pancreas and increases sensitivity of tissues to insulin
Contraindications	Diabetic ketoacidosis, cardiovascular disease
Side Effects	Dizziness, headache, nausea, decreased B_{12} absorption (metformin)
Special Instructions	Take with breakfast or first main meal
Drug Interactions	Furosemide and nifedipine (metformin)

Examples: Hypoglycemic Agents				
Generic Name	**Dosage**	**Dosage Form**	**Hypoglycemic Class**	**Indication**
Canagliflozin	100 mg PO QD	Tablet	SGLT-2 Inhibitor	Adjunct to diet and exercise for type II diabetes, and reduce risk of cardiovascular death in adults with type II diabetes
Glimepiride	1 mg–4 mg PO QD, max daily dose of 8 mg	Tablet	Sulfonylurea (2nd generation)	Adjunct to diet and exercise for type II diabetes, for use in combination with insulin to lower blood glucose
Glipizide	5 mg–20 mg PO QD, max daily dose of 40 mg	Tablet	Sulfonylurea (2nd generation)	Adjunct to diet and exercise for type II diabetes
Glyburide	2.5 mg–5 mg PO QD/BID, max dose is 20 mg/day	Tablet	Sulfonylurea (2nd generation)	Adjunct to diet and exercise for type II diabetes
Linagliptin	5 mg PO QD	Tablet	DPP-4 Inhibitor	Adjunct to diet and exercise for type II diabetes

Examples: Hypoglycemic Agents

Generic Name	Dosage	Dosage Form	Hypoglycemic Class	Indication
Liraglutide	1.2 mg SC QD, may increase to 1.8 mg	Injection	GLP-1 Agonist	Adjunct to diet and exercise for type II diabetes, and reduce risk of cardiovascular death in adults with type II diabetes
Metformin	500 mg PO BID, may increase up to maximum daily dose of 2550 mg	Tablet	Biguanide	Adjunct to diet and exercise for type II diabetes
Pioglitazone	15 mg–30 mg PO QD, up to 45 mg PO QD	Tablet	Glitazone	Adjunct to diet and exercise for type II diabetes
Sitagliptin	100 mg PO QD	Tablet	DPP-4 inhibitor	Adjunct to diet and exercise for type II diabetes

Combination Hypoglycemic Agents

Generic Name	Dosage	Dosage Form	Indication
Sitagliptin and Metformin	50 mg sitagliptin/ 1000 mg metformin to 100 mg sitagliptin/ 1000 mg metformin PO QD	Tablet	Adjunct to diet and exercise for type II diabetes

DRUG CLASS: INSULIN			
Mechanism of Action	Lowers blood glucose levels by stimulating glucose uptake and by inhibiting glucose production		
Contraindications	Hypoglycemia		
Side Effects	Hypoglycemia, redness and swelling at injection site		
Special Instructions	Doses of insulin are highly individualized		
Drug Interactions	Corticosteroids, diltiazem, epinephrine, oral contraceptives, beta blockers		
Examples: Insulin			
Generic Name	**Dosage**	**Dosage Form**	**Indication**
Insulin glargine	Injection	Long-Acting	Treatment of type I and type II diabetes
Insulin human	Injection	Intermediate	Treatment of type I and type II diabetes
Insulin aspart	Injection	Fast-Acting	Treatment of type I and type II diabetes
Insulin detemir	Injection	Long-Acting	Treatment of type I and type II diabetes

DRUG CLASS: BISPHOSPHONATES	
Mechanism of Action	Adheres to osteoclasts (breaks down bone) to prevent bone resorption
Contraindications	Esophageal abnormalities, patients who cannot sit upright or stand for 30 minutes
Side Effects	Abdominal pain, constipation, flatulence
Special Instructions	Must be swallowed with 8 ounces plain water immediately after rising for the day and must be 30 minutes before first food, beverage or medication of the day
Drug Interactions	Calcium and antacids, aspirin

Examples: Bisphosphonates

Generic Name	Dosage	Dosage Form	Indication
Alendronate	10 mg PO QD or 70 mg PO QWEEK	Tablet	Treatment and prevention of osteoporosis in postmenopausal women
Ibandronate (Boniva)	150 mg PO QWEEKS or 3 mg IV over 15–30 seconds	Tablet Injection	Treatment and prevention of osteoporosis in postmenopausal women
Risderonate (Actonel)	5 mg PO QD 35 mg PO QWEEK 150 mg PO QMONTH	Tablet	Treatment and prevention of osteoporosis in postmenopausal women, osteoporosis in men
Zoledronic acid (Zometa)	5 mg IV infused over 15 minutes every 2 years	Injection	Treatment and prevention of osteoporosis in postmenopausal women

DRUG CLASS: ANDROGENS	
Mechanism of Action	Activates androgen receptors
Contraindications	Breast or prostate cancer, high cholesterol, liver problems
Side Effects	Headache, anxiety, facial hair growth, numbness or tingling
Special Instructions	Testosterone is a Schedule III medication
Drug Interactions	Warfarin

Example: Androgen			
Generic Name	**Dosage**	**Dosage Form**	**Indication**
Testosterone	50 mg–400 mg IM Q4W	Injection	Deficiency of testosterone, hypogonadism

DRUG CLASS: ORAL CONTRACEPTIVES	
Mechanism of Action	Suppresses LH and FSH, resulting in inhibition of ovulation
Contraindications	Clotting disorders, pregnancy, breast cancer
Side Effects	Abdominal cramping, acne edema
Special Instructions	Intended to prevent pregnancy; does not protect against sexually transmitted diseases
Drug Interactions	Antibiotics may alter absorption; St. John's wort may reduce effectiveness

Examples: Oral Contraceptives			
Generic Name	**Dosage**	**Dosage Form**	**Indication**
Ethinyl estradiol and desogestrel	1 tab PO QD × 21 or 28 days	Tablet	Prevention of pregnancy
Ethinyl estradiol and drospirenone	1 tab PO QD × 28 days	Tablet	Prevention of pregnancy
Ethinyl estradiol and levonorgestrel	1 tab PO QD × 21 or 28 days	Tablet	Prevention of pregnancy
Ethinyl estradiol and norethindrone	1 tab PO QD × 21 or 28 days	Tablet	Prevention of pregnancy
Ethinyl estradiol and norgestimate	1 tab PO QD × 28 days	Tablet	Prevention of pregnancy

DRUG CLASS: HORMONE REPLACEMENT THERAPY	
Mechanism of Action	Acts on estrogen receptors
Contraindications	Genital bleeding, breast cancer, DVT, PE
Side Effects	Abnormal menstrual bleeding, edema, changes in weight, mental depression, insomnia
Special Instructions	Must be discontinued if pregnancy occurs
Drug Interactions	Antibiotics may alter absorption, St. John's Wort

Examples: Hormone Replacement Therapy			
Generic Name	Dosage	Dosage Form	Indication
Estradiol	1 mg–2 mg PO QD	Tablet	Treatment of moderate to severe vasomotor symptoms associated with menopause
Conjugated estrogens	1.25 mg PO QD	Tablet Vaginal cream Injection	Treatment of moderate to severe vasomotor symptoms associated with menopause, prostatic carcinoma
Ethinyl estradiol and norethindrone	1 tab PO QD	Tablet	Treatment of moderate to severe vasomotor symptoms associated with menopause, prevention of osteoporosis

DRUG CLASS: PROGESTIN HORMONES	
Mechanism of Action	Prevention of ovulation
Contraindications	Peanut allergy, known or suspected pregnancy, may worsen depression
Side Effects	Dizziness, headache, abdominal pain, blurred or loss of vision
Special Instructions	May be taken with milk or food in case of upset stomach
Drug Interactions	Ketoconazole

Example: Progestin Hormones			
Generic Name	Dosage	Dosage Form	Indication
Progesterone	200 mg PO QPM × 12 days in a 28-day cycle	Capsule	Endometrial hyperplasia; signs and symptoms of secondary amenorrhea

The Muscles and Joints

A joint is a union between two or more bones. There are several different types of joints, including **hinge joints** (elbows, ankles, and knees), **ball-and-socket joints** (shoulders and hips), and **pivot joints** (vertebrae and neck). Joints are surrounded by fluid (synovial) to allow gliding movement. A **bursa** is a sac containing synovial fluid. **Ligaments** surround and reinforce a joint and connect a joint to a bone.

Muscles allow joints and bones to move by contracting to produce movement. A **tendon** connects a muscle to a bone. There are three types of muscle: skeletal, smooth, and cardiac. **Skeletal** muscle is voluntary—used to consciously control movement. **Smooth** muscle is involuntary and is found in the lining of organs such as the stomach or intestines. **Involuntary** muscles contract without conscious control. **Cardiac** muscle is found in the heart and is also involuntary. Bones, joints, and muscles work together to allow movement of the body.

Disorders of Muscles and Joints

Disorder	Description
Muscle Spasm	Involuntary muscle contractions
Inflammation	Reddening, swelling, and hot; often as a result of injury or infection
Fever	Abnormally high body temperature, often treated with medications used for pain and inflammation; antipyretic reduces fever
Pain	Physical discomfort caused by illness or injury; treated with analgesic
Arthritis	Inflammation of the joints

Drug classes used to treat disorders of the muscles and joints include the following:

- Muscle relaxants
- Non-steroidal anti-inflammatory drugs (NSAIDs)
- Cyclooxygenase-2 (COX-2) inhibitors
- Nonnarcotic analgesics
- Narcotic analgesics
- Antirheumatic agents

DRUG CLASS: MUSCLE RELAXANTS	
Mechanism of Action	Exact mechanism is unknown but is a CNS depressant and causes sedation
Contraindications	Renal or liver impairment, patients with CHF (cyclobenzaprine)
Side Effects	Drowsiness, dizziness, dry mouth, fatigue, blurred vision, rash
Special Instructions	May cause drowsiness, use caution when operating machinery
Drug Interactions	Other CNS depressants, including alcohol

Examples: Muscle Relaxants			
Generic Name	**Dosage**	**Dosage Form**	**Indication**
Carisoprodol	250 mg–350 mg PO TID and HS	Tablet	Relief of discomfort associated with musculoskeletal conditions
Cyclobenzaprine	5 mg PO TID can increase to 10 mg TID	Tablet Capsule	Relief of skeletal muscle spasm
Methocarbamol	750 mg–1000 mg PO QID	Tablet	As an adjunct to rest and physical therapy for the relief of acute painful musculoskeletal conditions
	30 mL Infused or IM maximum per day	Injection	

DRUG CLASS: NSAIDS	
Mechanism of Action	Inhibits cyclooxygenase, which causes a decrease in prostaglandin production and lowers inflammation; NSAIDs produce antipyretic, anti-inflammatory, and analgesic effects
Contraindications	GI toxicity such as bleeding, ulcers, or perforation; pregnancy
Side Effects	Nausea, indigestion, constipation, heartburn, tinnitus; administering aspirin to children may cause Reye's syndrome, a rare but serious condition causing liver damage and brain swelling
Special Instructions	May take with food or milk in case of GI upset
Drug Interactions	Aspirin, loop diuretics, lithium, beta blockers, warfarin

Examples: NSAIDs			
Generic Name	**Dosage**	**Dosage Form**	**Indication**
Aspirin*	OTC therapy started at 81 mg PO QD	Tablet	Inflammation, fever, and pain
Diclofenac	50 mg PO TID/QID, 75 mg PO BID, or 100 mg PO QD/BID	Tablet (extended release) Tablet (enteric-coated)	Rheumatoid arthritis, osteoarthritis, ankylosing spondylitis
Ibuprofen*	600 mg–800 mg PO TID/QID	Tablet	Mild to moderate pain, dysmenorrhea, rheumatoid arthritis and osteoarthritis
Meloxicam	7.5 mg PO QD, can increase to 15 mg	Tablet Oral suspension	Rheumatoid arthritis, osteoarthritis
Naproxen*	275 mg PO Q6–8 HOURS PRN	Tablet	Mild to moderate pain, rheumatoid arthritis, osteoarthritis, relief of acute gout

* sold OTC

Drug Class: COX-2 Inhibitor	
Mechanism of Action	Inhibits cyclooxygenase-2 (COX-2), which produces prostaglandins; this leads to reduced levels of inflammation. COX-2 inhibitors are antipyretic, anti-inflammatory, and analgesic
Contraindications	Patients who are allergic or sensitive to NSAIDs, ulcer or gastrointestinal disease, pregnancy
Side Effects	Diarrhea, dyspepsia, abdominal pain
Special Instructions	May be taken with food if necessary
Drug Interactions	May decrease effect of ACE inhibitors, lithium warfarin

Example: COX-2 Inhibitor			
Generic Name	**Dosage**	**Dosage Form**	**Indication**
Celecoxib	200 mg PO QD or 100 mg PO BID	Capsule	Rheumatoid arthritis, osteoarthritis, management of acute pain, and dysmenorrhea

DRUG CLASS: NONNARCOTIC ANALGESICS	
Mechanism of Action	Acetaminophen inhibits prostaglandins, which leads to antipyretic and analgesic effects
Contraindications	Renal and liver impairment
Side Effects	Nausea, cramping, liver toxicity
Special Instructions	It is important to stay under 3000 mg/day when taking acetaminophen; chronic use over 3000 mg may cause liver damage
Drug Interactions	Warfarin, carbamazepine, phenytoin

Examples: Nonnarcotic Analgesics			
Generic Name	**Dosage**	**Dosage Form**	**Indication**
Acetaminophen*	325 mg–650 mg PO Q4H PRN—must not exceed 3,000 mg/day (4,000 mg/day under medical supervision)	Tablet Caplet Caplet (extended release) Oral liquid Oral suspension Tablet (chewable) Injection	Mild to moderate pain, osteoarthritis, fever

* sold OTC

DRUG CLASS: NARCOTIC ANALGESICS	
Mechanism of Action	Block pain impulse in CNS
Contraindications	Pulmonary disease, hepatic and renal impairment
Side Effects	Dizziness, drowsiness, constipation, nausea and vomiting, respiratory depression
Special Instructions	Avoid alcohol, may be habit forming
Drug Interactions	Other CNS depressants and alcohol, MAOIs and TCAs

Examples: Narcotic Analgesics			
Generic Name	**Dosage**	**Dosage Form**	**Indication**
Acetaminophen with hydrocodone	One to two tablets or 3 teaspoonsful PO Q4–6 HOURS PRN PAIN	Tablet Elixir	Moderate to severe pain
Hydrocodone	20 mg PO QD	Tablet (extended release)	Severe pain
Morphine	15 mg–200 mg PO Q12 HOURS	Tablet	Moderate to severe pain
Oxycodone	10 mg–20 mg PO BID	Tablet (controlled release)	Moderate to severe pain when using an opiate for longer period is tolerated
Tramadol	50 mg–100 mg PO Q4–6 HOURS, max dose is 400 mg/day	Tablet Tablet (extended release)	Moderate to severe pain

DRUG CLASS: ANTIRHEUMATIC AGENTS	
Mechanism of Action	Mechanism is unknown
Contraindications	Pregnancy, liver disease, retinopathy
Side Effects	Headache, visual disturbances, weight loss
Special Instructions	Take with food or milk for upset stomach
Drug Interactions	NSAIDs (methotrexate)

Examples: Antirheumatic Agents			
Generic Name	**Dosage**	**Dosage Form**	**Indication**
Hydroxychloroquine	400 mg–600 mg PO QD	Tablet	Rheumatoid arthritis, malaria
Methotrexate	10 mg–25 mg PO Per week	Tablet Injection	Treatment of breast cancer, control of psoriasis, treatment of arthritis

Integumentary System

The integumentary system includes the skin, hair, and nails and protects the body from external damage and loss of water. The **epidermis** is the outer layer of the skin, and the **dermis** is directly below the epidermis. Some drugs are known to cause photosensitivity, which is an abnormal sensitivity to sunlight and can cause excessive burning.

Drugs that can cause photosensitivity include the following:

- Amiodarone
- Diltiazem
- Diphenhydramine
- Furosemide
- Hydrochlorothiazide
- Metformin
- Methotrexate
- Sertraline
- Simvastatin

Drug classes that are known to cause photosensitivity include the following:

- ACE inhibitors
- NSAIDs
- Sulfa antibiotics
- Tetracycline antibiotics
- TCAs

Disorders of the Skin

Disorder	Description
Eczema	Itchy, red, dry condition caused by inflammation
Acne	Infected sebaceous glands in the skin
Psoriasis	Chronic condition with patches of red, scaly skin; genetically linked; immune system is involved
Impetigo	Red sores around mouth and nose that may rupture, ooze and crust, highly infectious
Athlete's foot	Fungal infection occurs between the toes
Jock itch	Fungal infection in the skin between the buttocks, groin, and inner thighs
Ringworm	Fungal infection on the skin or scalp, highly contagious

Drug classes used to treat skin disorders include the following:

- Topical corticosteroids
- Retinoid
- Monoclonal antibody
- Topical antibiotic
- Topical antifungal

DRUG CLASS: TOPICAL CORTICOSTEROIDS			
Mechanism of Action	Prevents synthesis of inflammation mediators (prostaglandin and leukotriene)		
Contraindications	Should be used with caution in patients with dermatological infections		
Side Effects	Local burning and itching, skin atrophy		
Special Instructions	Do not use around the eyes; do not use for more than two consecutive weeks (clobetasol)		
Drug Interactions	Systemic corticosteroids		
Examples: Topical Corticosteroids			
Generic Name	**Dosage**	**Dosage Form**	**Indication**
Clobetasol	A thin film is applied BID–QID	Cream Gel Ointment Solution	Relief of inflammatory and pruritic manifestations of dermatoses
Hydrocortisone*	Apply to affected area BID–TID	Ointment Cream	Relief of inflammatory and pruritic manifestations of dermatoses
Triamcinolone	A thin film is applied BID–QID	Ointment Cream Lotion Aerosol Paste	Relief of inflammatory and pruritic manifestations of dermatoses; temporary relief of symptoms associated with oral inflammatory lesions

* sold OTC

DRUG CLASS: RETINOIDS	
Mechanism of Action	Impacts cell death and differentiation, leading to a reduction in sebum (oil secretion) production
Contraindications	Pregnancy; patients must demonstrate no pregnancy prior to beginning treatment, and must agree to use two forms of birth control while taking
Side Effects	Dry skin and lips, cracked corners of the mouth, nosebleeds, itching, rash
Special Instructions	Avoid prolonged exposure to sunlight, contact lenses may become dry and uncomfortable to wear during treatment
Drug Interactions	Doxycycline

Example: Retinoids			
Generic Name	**Dosage**	**Dosage Form**	**Indication**
Isotretinoin	20 mg PO QD	Capsule	Severe nodular acne

DRUG CLASS: MONOCLONAL ANTIBODY	
Mechanism of Action	Binds to tumor necrosis factor (TNF) and blocks interaction with receptors, this leads to decrease in inflammatory response
Contraindications	Active infections, tuberculosis, autoimmune disease
Side Effects	Headaches, nausea, pain at injection site, infections and immune reactions
Special Instructions	Must be refrigerated
Drug Interactions	Other biologic drugs such as DMARDs or monoclonal antibodies

Example: Monoclonal Antibody			
Generic Name	**Dosage**	**Dosage Form**	**Indication**
Adalimumab	40 mg/0.8 mL subcutaneously every other week	Injection	Psoriasis, Crohn's disease

DRUG CLASS: TOPICAL ANTIBIOTIC	
Mechanism of Action	Inhibits bacterial protein synthesis
Contraindications	Ophthalmic use
Side Effects	Burning, stinging and pain, headache, rhinitis, congestion
Special Instructions	Must be refrigerated
Drug Interactions	Other biologic drugs such as DMARDs or monoclonal antibodies

Example: Topical Antibiotic			
Generic Name	**Dosage**	**Dosage Form**	**Indication**
Mupirocin	Cover area with a small film TID	Ointment Nasal ointment Cream	Impetigo

DRUG CLASS: TOPICAL ANTIFUNGAL	
Mechanism of Action	Inhibits fungal cell wall synthesis
Contraindications	Pregnancy, children under 2 years old
Side Effects	Burning, stinging at application site
Special Instructions	Should be discontinued immediately if blistering, severe redness, or peeling occurs
Drug Interactions	Warfarin

Examples: Topical Antifungal			
Generic Name	**Dosage**	**Dosage Form**	**Indication**
Clotrimazole (Lotrimin)*	Apply to affected area BID	Cream Spray	Athlete's foot, jock itch, ringworm
Terbinafine (Lamisil)*	Apply to affected area QD	Cream Gel Spray	Athlete's foot, jock itch, ringworm

* sold OTC

The Eye

Medications used to treat the eye are administered opthalmically. The eye is covered by a thick membrane known as the **conjunctiva**. The iris is the colored portion of the eye. The **pupil** is the dark circle in the middle of the eye that adjusts in response to light and allows the proper amount of light to enter the eye. The **lens** helps focus the image, and the **optic nerve** takes the image and sends the message to the brain.

Disorders of the Eye

Disorder	Description
Glaucoma	Chronic high internal pressure in the eye which can destroy the optic nerve and cause blindness
Conjunctivitis	Also known as pink eye, inflammation of the membrane in the eyelid and outside of the eyeball; treated with ophthalmic antibiotics

DRUGS USED TO TREAT GLAUCOMA	
Mechanism of Action	Reduces flow of aqueous humor production or increases the outflow of aqueous humor, which reduces intraocular pressure
Contraindications	Patients with depression, coronary insufficiency, asthma, taste perversion, and burning (dorzolamide and timolol)
Side Effects	eye pruritis, allergic conjunctivitis
Special Instructions	Avoid squinting or closing eyes tightly after instilling drops
Drug Interactions	MAOIs, TCAs, additive effects may occur if given with beta blockers

Examples: Drugs Used to Treat Glaucoma			
Generic Name	Dosage	Dosage Form	Indication
Brimonidine	One drop into affected eye TID (8 hours apart)	Ophthalmic solution	Reduction of intraocular pressure in patients with glaucoma or ocular hypertension
Dorzolamide and timolol	One drop into affected eye BID	Ophthalmic solution	Reduction of intraocular pressure in patients with glaucoma or ocular hypertension
Latanoprost	One drop into affected eye QPM	Ophthalmic solution	Reduction of intraocular pressure in patients with glaucoma or ocular hypertension
Timolol	One drop into affected eye BID	Ophthalmic solution	Reduction of intraocular pressure in patients with glaucoma or ocular hypertension

ANTIBIOTICS FOR EYE INFECTIONS	
Mechanism of Action	Prevents growth of bacteria on the eye
Contraindications	Contact lenses, fungal and viral infections
Side Effects	Stinging, burning, itching, and redness of the eye after administration, eyelid itching and crusting
Special Instructions	Warm the tube by holding in hand prior to administration, do not touch applicator tip to eye
Drug Interactions	Furosemide, bumetanide

Examples: Antibiotics for Eye Infections			
Generic Name	**Dosage**	**Dosage Form**	**Indication**
Bacitracin; Neomycin; Polymyxin B	Apply a thin strip to affected eye every 3–4 hours for 7–10 days	Ophthalmic ointment	Treatment of ophthalmic infection caused by bacteria
Erythromycin	Apply a thin strip to affected eye up to 6 times daily	Ophthalmic ointment	Treatment of ophthalmic infection caused by bacteria

The Ear

The ear is composed of an inner, middle, and outer structure. Sound is processed through the ear canal and ends at the ear drum (tympanic membrane). The ear can accumulate wax and cause a buildup, pain, or loss of hearing. This is generally treated with OTC wax dissolvers such as carbamide peroxide (Debrox). The ear can also become infected, known as an earache or otitis media. An ear infection is treated with antibiotic ear drops administered otically.

The Immune System

The immune system is the mechanism of defense for our body against foreign substances. **T-cells** are white blood cells (lymphocytes) that help maintain immunity. **White blood cells** are produced in the bone marrow. The **thymus** helps mature and generate T-cells. **Lymph nodes** throughout the body create a network of fluid and filters that catch foreign substances. The **spleen** also acts as a filter, removing dead red blood cells and storing white blood cells and platelets.

Disorders of the Immune System

Disorder	Description
Bacterial Infection	An infection caused by bacteria when the body's immune system cannot fight off the bacteria
Fungal Infection	An infection caused by a fungus that occurs systemically in immunocompromised patients; topical fungal infections grow in dark, warm, moist locations such as the bottom of the feet or groin
Viral Infection	An infection caused by a virus usually through direct contact or inhalation of particles; can be acute or chronic and symptoms are generally more severe than bacterial infection

Drug classes used to treat infections include the following:

- Antibiotics
  - Penicillins
  - Macrolides
  - Fluoroquinolones
  - Cephalosporins
  - Tetracyclines
  - Sulfonamides
  - Other Antimicrobials
- Antiviral Agents
- Antifungal Agents

DRUG CLASS: PENICILLIN ANTIBIOTICS	
Mechanism of Action	Inhibits the synthesis of the bacterial cell wall and kills the bacteria (bactericidal)
Contraindications	Renal impairment, cephalosporin allergy (cross-sensitivity is 5–10%)
Side Effects	Nausea, vomiting, diarrhea, rash, itching
Special Instructions	Take on an empty stomach, complete full course of therapy
Drug Interactions	Oral contraceptives

Examples: Penicillin Antibiotics			
Generic Name	**Dosage**	**Dosage Form**	**Indication**
Amoxicillin	250 mg–500 mg PO Q8H or 500 mg–875 mg PO Q12H	Tablet Tablet (chewable) Capsule Oral suspension	Infections caused by gram-negative organisms, gonorrhea
Amoxicillin and clavulanate	500 mg amoxicillin/125 mg clavulanate tablet PO Q8H or 875 mg amoxicillin/125 mg clavulanate tablet PO Q12H	Tablet Tablet (chewable) Tablet (extended release) Oral suspension	Sinusitis, otitis media, community-acquired pneumonia, skin infections, UTI

Drug Class: Macrolide Antibiotics	
Mechanism of Action	Prevents bacterial protein synthesis, which stops bacterial growth (bacteriostatic)
Contraindications	Liver impairment, complicated pneumonia, gonorrhea, and syphilis
Side Effects	Diarrhea, nausea, vomiting, abdominal pain
Special Instructions	Do not take antacids within one hour of administration, take on an empty stomach
Drug Interactions	Antacids

Examples: Macrolide Antibiotics			
Generic Name	**Dosage**	**Dosage Form**	**Indication**
Azithromycin	500 mg on first day, then 250 mg once daily for 4 days (ZPAK)	Tablet Oral suspension Injection	Infections of the lower and upper respiratory tract, skin infections
Clarithromycin	1000 mg PO QD × 7–14 days	Tablet Tablet (extended release) Oral suspension	Pharyngitis, tonsillitis, sinusitis, bronchitis, pneumonia, community-acquired pneumonia, otitis media, skin infections

DRUG CLASS: FLUOROQUINOLONE ANTIBIOTICS	
Mechanism of Action	Prevents bacterial DNA synthesis, which kills the bacteria (bactericidal)
Contraindications	May cause ruptures in shoulder, hand, and Achilles tendons (black box warning), must be discontinued at first sign of rash
Side Effects	Nausea, rash, diarrhea, photosensitivity, dizziness
Special Instructions	Take all medication until therapy completed, avoid excessive periods of sun
Drug Interactions	Antacids, NSAIDs, warfarin

Examples: Fluoroquinolone Antibiotics

Generic Name	Dosage	Dosage Form	Indication
Ciprofloxacin	250 mg–500 mg PO Q12H	Tablet Tablet (extended release) Oral suspension Injection	Infectious diarrhea, respiratory tract infections, cystitis, UTI, gonorrhea
Levofloxacin	500 mg PO QD × 7 days	Tablet Oral solution Injection	Bronchitis, pneumonia, UTI, anthrax

DRUG CLASS: CEPHALOSPORIN ANTIBIOTICS	
Mechanism of Action	Inhibits the synthesis of the bacterial cell wall and kills the bacteria (bactericidal)
Contraindications	Hypersensitivity to penicillin (cross-sensitivity is 5–10%)
Side Effects	Nausea, vomiting, diarrhea, hives, itching, and rash
Special Instructions	Take on empty stomach at even intervals, complete full course of therapy
Drug Interactions	Oral contraceptives

Examples: Cephalosporin Antibiotics

Generic Name	Dosage	Dosage Form	Indication
Cephalexin	250 mg–1000 mg PO Q6H	Capsule Tablet Oral suspension	Cystitis, infections due to *E. coli*, streptococci, staphylococci, *H. influenzae*
Cefdinir	600 mg PO daily in one or two doses	Capsule Oral suspension	Community-acquired pneumonia, pharyngitis, tonsillitis, skin infection, otitis media

DRUG CLASS: TETRACYCLINE ANTIBIOTICS	
Mechanism of Action	Prevents bacterial protein synthesis, which stops bacterial growth (bacteriostatic)
Contraindications	Should not be used in children under eight years old (causes permanent stains on teeth)
Side Effects	Dizziness, vertigo, photosensitivity, sore or darkened tongue
Special Instructions	Taken on empty stomach, complete full course of therapy, avoid sunlight
Drug Interactions	Oral contraceptives, digoxin, antacids

Examples: Tetracycline Antibiotics			
Generic Name	**Dosage**	**Dosage Form**	**Indication**
Doxycycline	100 mg PO Q12H	Tablet Capsule Oral syrup Oral suspension Injection	Gram negative bacterial infections, syphilis, gonorrhea, chlamydia
Tetracycline	250 mg–500 mg PO BID–QID	Capsule	Gram negative bacterial infections, syphilis, gonorrhea, chlamydia, acne

DRUG CLASS: SULFONAMIDE ANTIBIOTICS	
Mechanism of Action	Inhibits para-aminobenzoic acid (PABA), which is a required growth factor in bacterial cells, and prevents growth (bacteriostatic)
Contraindications	Infants less than two months old, pregnancy and nursing, renal and liver impairment
Side Effects	Photosensitivity, nausea, vomiting, diarrhea, dizziness, rash
Special Instructions	Take on empty stomach, complete full course of therapy, avoid sunlight
Drug Interactions	Warfarin

Example: Sulfonamide Antibiotics			
Generic Name	**Dosage**	**Dosage Form**	**Indication**
Sulfamethoxazole and trimethoprim	800 mg sulfamethoxazole / 160 mg trimethoprim Q12H × 10–14 days	Tablet (regular strength) Tablet (double strength) Oral suspension Injection	UTI, otitis media

Examples: Other Antimicrobials

Generic Name	Dosage	Dosage Form	Indication
Metronidazole	250 mg–500 mg PO TID × 7 days	Tablet Capsule Tablet (extended release) Injection	Bacterial vaginosis, trichomoniasis
Clindamycin	150 mg–450 mg PO Q6H	Capsule	Respiratory tract infections, skin and intra-abdominal infections, infections of genital tract
Nitrofurantoin	100 mg PO Q12H × 7 days	Capsule Capsule (macrocrystal) Suspension	UTI

DRUG CLASS: ANTIVIRALS

Mechanism of Action	Inhibits viral DNA to prevent outbreaks
Contraindications	Renal impairment, dehydrated patients (may form kidney stones)
Side Effects	Nausea, vomiting, headache, abdominal pain
Special Instructions	Should drink plenty of water to avoid kidney stone formation
Drug Interactions	Probenecid

Examples: Antivirals

Generic Name	Dosage	Dosage Form	Indication
Acyclovir	200 mg PO Q4H, 5 times daily × 10 days	Capsule Tablet Ointment Cream Oral suspension Injection	Genital herpes, treatment for chickenpox, treatment of herpes zoster (shingles)
Valacyclovir	1 gram PO BID × 10 days	Tablet	Genital herpes, treatment of herpes zoster (shingles), treatment of cold sores

DRUG CLASS: ORAL ANTIFUNGALS	
Mechanism of Action	Inhibits fungal enzymes, which inhibits fungal growth
Contraindications	Liver impairment, patients with arrhythmia, pregnancy and nursing
Side Effects	Nausea, headache, abdominal pain, diarrhea, dizziness
Special Instructions	Tablet should be protected from light
Drug Interactions	Warfarin, phenytoin, glipizide

Example: Oral Antifungals			
Generic Name	**Dosage**	**Dosage Form**	**Indication**
Fluconazole	150 mg PO one dose	Tablet Oral suspension Injection	Vaginal candidiasis (yeast infection), esophageal candidiasis, oropharyngeal candidiasis

Vitamins, Minerals, Electrolytes, and Supplements

Vitamins are organic substances required for normal body function. The body does not make vitamins, so we rely on a healthy diet to prevent any vitamin deficiencies. There are two types of vitamins: water-soluble and fat-soluble. **Water-soluble vitamins** are excreted from the kidneys more easily then **fat-soluble vitamins**. Below are the vitamins and essential functions and indications for each.

Vitamin	Generic Name	Function	Soluble
A	Retinol	Promotes good vision, maintains healthy teeth and skin	Fat
B_1	Thiamine	Releases energy from carbohydrates during metabolism	Water
B_2	Riboflavin	Releases energy from protein, fat, and carbohydrates during metabolism	Water
B_3	Niacin	Releases energy from protein, fat, and carbohydrates during metabolism	Water
B_5	Pantothenic acid	Makes blood cells and releases energy from protein, fat, and carbohydrates	Water
B_6	Pyridoxine	Builds tissues and metabolism of protein	Water
B_7	Biotin	Releases energy from protein, fat, and carbohydrates during metabolism	Water
B_9	Folic Acid	Genetic material development and red blood cell production, important to take during pregnancy	Water
B_{12}	Cyanocobalamin	Cell development and metabolism of fat and protein	Water
C	Ascorbic Acid	Growth and repair of tissues, wound healing	Water
D_2	Ergocalciferol	Helps body absorb calcium and phosphorus	Fat
D_3	Cholecalciferol	Helps body absorb calcium and phosphorus	Fat
E	Tocopherols	Antioxidant	Fat
K	Phytonadione	Blood clotting	Fat

Minerals are necessary for proper functioning of many processes in the body. **Electrolytes** are minerals which have an ionic charge associated with them. Below are electrolytes and their function.

Mineral	Function
Calcium	Bone growth and prevention of osteoporosis
Sodium	Nerve impulses and muscle contractions, water regulation
Potassium	Nerve impulses and muscle contractions, water regulation
Chloride	Maintains blood pressure, blood volume, and pH of body fluids
Iron	Red blood cell production
Magnesium	Regulates heartbeat, blood glucose levels, and nerve and muscle function

Supplements are drugs manufactured to provide nutrients extracted from a plant (herbal) or synthetic sources to enhance the diet. There are many different types of supplements, and although the FDA requires safety testing, effectiveness does not have to be proven. It can also be dangerous for patients to self-medicate with herbal supplements and forego medication prescribed by a provider. There are some known interactions with prescription medications, but there is a lack of data, as these drugs to not undergo the same testing as prescription drugs.

Supplement	Uses
Aloe vera	Proper functioning of digestive system, wound and burn healing
Black cohosh	Menopausal symptoms and premenstrual syndrome
Chamomile	Sedative, calming agent
Chondroitin	Arthritis, often taken with glucosamine
Cinnamon	Lowers cholesterol, used for upset stomach
Cranberry	Urinary tract health
Coenzyme Q10	High blood pressure and high cholesterol
Dandelion	Loss of appetite, upset stomach, laxative
Echinacea	Immune system support
Feverfew	Prevention and treatment of migraines
Ginger	Nausea and motion sickness
Gingko	Cognitive function and memory
Ginseng	Boost energy, lower blood sugar, reduce cholesterol, reduce stress
Glucosamine	Arthritis, often taken with chondroitin
Kava	Anxiety, stress, and calming for insomnia
Melatonin	Insomnia
Milk thistle	Liver disease
Saw palmetto	BPH
St. John's wort	Depression
Valerian	Insomnia, anxiety

DRUG STABILITY

The **stability** of a drug is the length of time the product can retain its chemical, physical, and therapeutic properties. Many factors can affect drug stability, including pH, temperature, moisture, light, and potential incompatibilities. An **expiration date**, which indicates the length of time the drug will remain stable if stored under appropriate and specified conditions, is given to every manufactured medication. A **beyond-use date (BUD)**, which is often noted as "do not use after" or "use before," is used when preparing medications for patients. BUDs in sterile compounding take into consideration drug sterility and stability information, and the appropriate dating can be found in USP <797>.

Oral Suspensions

Drug stability can also depend on the dosage form of the medication. Oral suspensions prior to reconstitution will have an expiration date from the manufacturer on the label. After reconstitution, the BUD is reached in a substantially shorter time period. Stability is also dictated by proper temperature storage. Many oral suspensions can be stored at room temperature, but some must be refrigerated. Improper storage conditions can cause degradation of the drug and reduce effectiveness. Below are commonly prescribed oral suspensions and stability information after reconstitution.

Drug	Stability	Storage
Amoxicillin	14 days	Room temperature or refrigerated
Amoxicillin with clavulanate	10 days	Refrigerated
Azithromycin	10 days	Room temperature or refrigerated
Cephalexin	14 days	Refrigerated
Cefdinir	10 days	Room temperature or refrigerated
Clarithromycin	14 days	Room temperature
Penicillin VK	14 days	Refrigerated

Insulin

Stability of insulin is dependent on the type of insulin and storage conditions. Most insulin is stable for 28 days after opening, though there are a few types of insulin that are stable for 42 days after opening. If a vial of insulin is stored in the refrigerator and has not been opened, the expiration date on the manufacturer label is still valid. If an insulin vial or pen is found frozen, it should be discarded.

Below are commonly prescribed insulin (vials) and dating for stability after opening. It is important to note, the insulin listed below has the same dating if stored at room temperature or refrigerated after opening. The stability of many insulin pens is also 28 days after opening but varies based on insulin type.

Insulin	Stability after Opening
Insulin aspart (Novolog)	28 days
Insulin lispro (Humalog)	28 days
Insulin glulisine (Apidra)	28 days
Insulin regular (Humulin R)	28 days
Humulin N	28 days
Humulin 70/30	28 days
Humalog 75/25	28 days
Humalog 50/50	28 days
Novolog 70/30	28 days
Insulin glargine (Lantus)	28 days
Insulin detemir (Levemir)	42 days
Insulin regular (Novolin R)	42 days
Novolin N	42 days
Novolin 70/30	42 days

Reconstitutables

Many drugs are produced in a powder form because they degrade rapidly once in solution. These must be administered following reconstitution and are stable for only a brief period of time. **Reconstitution** is the process of combining a **diluent** (inactive liquid used to dilute or reconstitute a medication) with a powder to make a liquid solution. To ensure stability of the product, it is essential the correct diluent is used to reconstitute. Each vial will indicate the diluent on the label or package insert; sterile water or sodium chloride is often used to reconstitute medications. The volume used to reconstitute is also indicated on the label.

Stability of a drug after reconstitution is dependent on the medication. Some drugs are stable for a short period of time following reconstitution, while others may be stable for a few days. It is important to read the package insert or manufacturer label prior to reconstitution to determine the BUD for the reconstituted medication.

Injectables

Stability of injectable drugs that are already in solution depends on the presence of preservatives. A **single-dose vial (SDV)** or a single-use vial is intended for an injection or infusion that is generally reserved for a single patient or procedure. SDVs generally do not contain a preservative, as they are designed for one-time use. An SDV should be used for only one patient to prevent any contamination or outbreaks to other patients using the same vial. There may be times when an SDV can be used more than once for the same patient (for example, if a provider is titrating a dose). If the vial was opened within an ISO class 5 hood or isolator, the remaining contents are good for six hours after opening. An SDV is designed for one entry only, however, so if used again, a new needle and syringe should be used.

An **ampule** is also designated as single-use, as it does not contain preservatives. An ampule is a glass container that is opened by breaking the neck and removing contents with a filter needle. When an ampule is opened, it has a limited amount of stability remaining, as the contents of the ampule are now exposed to air. An ampule must be treated as a single-use and single-patient container when compounding.

Multi-dose vials (MDVs) contain more than one dose of medication in solution along with a preservative to help prevent the growth of a microbial. MDVs can be used on more than one patient, but the dose must be drawn up outside of patient treatment areas. Patient treatment areas include anywhere patients may be treated, such as operating rooms, procedure rooms, or patient rooms. If an MDV is opened in a patient treatment area, the infection from the patient area could contaminate the vial when a needle is inserted. This could potentially spread the infection to multiple patients. Once an MDV has been opened, it is stable for 28 days unless a different date is specified by the manufacturer. It is important to note that the expiration date must always be labeled on an MDV, NOT the date the vial was opened. This is often confused in practice, and for consistency, the expiration date should always be labeled.

Vaccinations

Vaccines are packaged in different dosage forms, including multi-dose vials, single-dose syringes or vials, and reconstitutable vials. If the vaccine is stored properly, single-dose syringes and vials are stable until reaching the expiration date listed on the drug label by the manufacturer. An opened MDV of vaccine that has been stored appropriately can also be used through the expiration date printed on the label, unless the manufacturer has established an earlier BUD. Many vaccines that specify an earlier BUD once opened are indicated to discard after 28 days. It is important to always check the vaccine package insert to determine if the vaccine has a BUD and for how long it can be stored after needle entry. Any vaccine not used prior to the BUD must be discarded.

For reconstituted vaccines, there are various requirements for stability. Some vaccine package inserts require the vaccine be discarded anywhere from immediately following reconstitution to 24 hours later. A vaccine with an immediate BUD must be reconstituted just prior to administration. For example, the rabies vaccine requires immediate administration after reconstitution, and stability will be limited if it is administered beyond this BUD.

Below are a few commonly administered vaccines and BUDs (assuming appropriate storage conditions).

Vaccine	Dosage Form	BUD
Rabies vaccine	Reconstitution	Immediately after reconstitution
Herpes zoster vaccine	Reconstitution	6 hours after reconstitution
Influenza vaccine	Multi-dose vial	28 days after opening
Varicella vaccine	Reconstitution	30 minutes after reconstitution
Tetanus, diphtheria, and pertussis vaccine	Single-dose syringe	Manufacturer expiration date
Pneumovax 23	Multi-dose vials	Manufacturer expiration date

NARROW THERAPEUTIC INDEX (NTI) MEDICATIONS

A **therapeutic index** is the dose, or range of doses, of a drug that is most effective without adverse events. Drugs that have a **narrow therapeutic index (NTI)** are those in which small differences in dosing may lead to a serious adverse reaction or therapeutic failure. The adverse reaction can lead to life-threatening injuries. Drugs that have a narrow therapeutic index may have requirements for generic substitution, as slight changes in bioequivalence may result in toxicity or ineffectiveness.

Below are frequently prescribed drugs with an NTI:

Generic	Brand	Drug Class
Carbamazepine	Tegretol	Antiepileptic
Digoxin	Digitek	Antiarrhythmic
Levothyroxine	Levoxyl, Levothroid	Thyroid hormone
Phenytoin	Dilantin	Antiepileptic
Warfarin	Coumadin	Anticoagulant

NTI medications have a small window between effective dose and toxicity. Often, these medications will cause serious complications if there is therapeutic failure. For example, many antiepileptic medications have an NTI. If the dosing is not precise, this could cause a patient to have uncontrolled seizures. Many times, prescribers will modify dosages in very small increments to avoid potential toxicity or adverse effects.

PHYSICAL AND CHEMICAL INCOMPATIBILITIES RELATED TO NON-STERILE COMPOUNDING AND RECONSTITUTION

During the compounding process, it is important to monitor for any signs of incompatibility. While a drug interaction happens within the body, an incompatibility occurs before drug administration, and is often visible. An incompatibility may occur when a drug reacts adversely with a compounding container, a solution or vehicle for mixing, or with another drug added into the compound.

One way to help prevent incompatibility is to review references for the proper diluent when reconstituting. For example, if the diluent needed is sodium chloride, and dextrose or water is used instead, this could risk an incompatibility with the powdered drug and diluent. In addition, when compounding non-sterile medications, it is essential to follow the master formula record for appropriate vehicle and container selection. Using Trissel's *Stability of Compounded Formulations* as a reference will help identify potential drug combinations that are not compatible.

There are two main types of incompatibility, physical and chemical.

Physical Incompatibility

Physical incompatibility results when two or more substances are mixed and a physical change occurs. This change could be in the form of a precipitate (solid formed from a solution), or a change in color, odor, taste, or viscosity (thickness). A common cause of physical incompatibility is a change in the pH level of the solution, or when a buffer is used that is not compatible with the drug.

Also considered a physical incompatibility is the reaction that may occur in an IV fluid bag or container. Most base solutions are produced in IV bags containing polyvinyl chloride (PVC). Some drugs interact with the PVC container, and this causes adsorption or adherence to the sides of the container. As a result, the medication will not be fully compounded or mixed, and the patient may not receive all of the medication in the infusion. For this reason, non-PVC IV bags or glass bottles or vials can be used to compound and administer these medications. Examples of medications that require non-PVC containers include insulin, nitroglycerin, and amiodarone.

Chemical Incompatibility

A **chemical incompatibility** occurs when a chemical reaction has caused a change in composition, which may include degradation or decomposition of the drug. Chemical reactions may be unnoticeable but may be observed through color or temperature change. The pH is often changed as well. As a result, the effectiveness of the drug may be reduced, which can cause harm to the patient or cause treatment to fail.

As one example of a chemical incompatibility, consider nitrogen tablets that have been repackaged in a bottle that is not resistant to light. Nitroglycerin is inactivated by light and moisture, and if the medication is degraded, a patient could risk serious harm through treatment failure.

PROPER STORAGE OF MEDICATIONS

All drugs have specific requirements for storage and handling. *The United States Pharmacopeia (USP)* defines storage requirements in USP Chapter <1079>. Starting at the manufacturing process, and through to patient administration, a drug must be stored properly to ensure stability.

Temperature Ranges

Storing medications within the proper temperature range is essential for drug effectiveness. The USP standards for temperature ranges are defined below:

Storage	Range (Celsius)	Range (Fahrenheit)
Freezer	–25°C to –10°C	–13°F to 14°F
Refrigerator (Cold)	2°C to 8°C	36°F to 46°F
Cool	8°C to 15°C	46°F to 59°F
Room Temperature	20°C to 25°C with excursions between 15°C and 30°C	68°F to 77°F with excursions between 59°F to 86°F
Warm	30°C to 40°C	86°F to 104°F

Vaccines are an important subset of medications that are most often refrigerated, but some may require freezing. Vaccines must be stored in refrigerators which are not the dormitory-style (medical grade only), and should not be stored on the top shelf or floor of the refrigerator. Refrigerated vaccines must never be stored in the freezer.

The following vaccines must be refrigerated and not frozen:

- Hepatitis A
- Hepatitis B
- HPV (human papillomavirus)
- Influenza
- Polio
- Meningococcal
- MMR (can also be kept frozen)
- Pneumococcal
- Rotavirus
- DTaP (pediatric diphtheria, tetanus, pertussis)
- TDAP (tetanus, diphtheria, and pertussis)
- Zoster

Live vaccines must be stored frozen. This includes the varicella (chicken pox) vaccine.

Consistent temperature monitoring is important to identify any temperature excursions and potential for loss of potency of drugs. Temperature recordings must be logged twice daily for any freezer or refrigerator containing a vaccine.

Light and Moisture Sensitivity

Additional storage restrictions include light and moisture sensitivity. Most outpatient prescription medication vials are amber in color to prevent light from degrading the medication inside. Some medications (such as nitroglycerin) are left in the original manufacturing packaging to protect from any light sensitivity.

If a medication is sensitive to moisture, it will be packaged with a desiccant inside the manufacturer stock bottle. A desiccant is used as a drying agent to absorb excess moisture and keep it from accumulating and damaging the stability of the drug. Medications packaged with a desiccant are often prepackaged in a 30-, 60-, or 90-count bottle, so the entire bottle can be dispensed for the prescription, keeping the desiccant in the bottle.

Restricted Access

In a hospital or institutional facility, certain medications may be accessible only to pharmacy staff, because these medications are not manufactured in their final dosage form and require compounding prior to patient administration.

Concentrated electrolytes must be diluted prior to administration. Some examples of concentrated electrolytes include the following:

- Hypertonic sodium chloride 3% (many facilities define as anything over 0.9%)
- Potassium chloride 2mEq/mL
- Magnesium sulfate 50%
- Sodium bicarbonate 8.4%
- Sodium chloride 23.4% solution

If these solutions are stocked on a nursing unit, a potentially harmful medication error will occur if these medications are administered prior to dilution.

An additional medication that must be stored only within the pharmacy is sterile water in 1000 mL bags used for injection, inhalation, or irrigation. The goal of restricting access to these bags is to prevent accidental infusion of sterile water to a patient. If a large volume of sterile water is infused, it can lead to significant patient harm or death. Sterile water is often used for respiratory therapy for ventilator patients and in surgery for reconstitution of dantrolene for treatment of malignant hyperthermia, so it is important to work with the appropriate departments when availability is limited.

Most facilities now utilize automated dispensing cabinets (ADCs) in nursing units to dispense medications for patient administration. Each of these cabinets is secure, and only authorized personnel may dispense medications from the cabinets. Nursing units may also have floor stock that includes frequently used medications, or diluents in a cupboard or cabinet. These medications are considered properly stored as long as they are not available to unauthorized individuals. This means the floor stock on each nursing unit must be continually monitored. If medications were stored in a laundry room or storage closet not near the nursing station, there would be a risk of unauthorized patients or individuals gaining access to these medications.

In both hospital and institutional settings, many chemotherapy and hazardous drugs are stored for patient use. Each of these medications is considered hazardous and be stored separately from other medications that are non-hazardous, including refrigerated products. USP Chapter <800> defines the storage requirements for hazardous drugs and will be discussed further in Chapter 4. Chapter 4 will also discuss storage of controlled substances, which require restricted access as well.

SUMMING IT UP

- **Pharmacology** is the study of the uses, effects, and mechanisms of action of drugs.

- Within pharmacology are two branches of study:

  1. **Pharmacodynamics** is the study of the effects of a drug on the body.

  2. **Pharmacokinetics** examines the movement of drug within the body during the absorption, distribution, metabolism, and elimination or excretion (ADME) processes.

     - **Absorption**, the first phase of a medication action, is the process of a drug entering the bloodstream.

     - Next the drug is distributed (**distribution**) from the blood to tissues and cells throughout the body.

     - **Metabolism**, the process of breaking down or converting the drug into a form that is more easily excreted, is next.

     - The final step, **elimination**, is the process of drug removal from the body.

- When a drug is approved by the FDA, it has three names:

  1. The **chemical name** of a drug is a complex description of the molecular structure and is generally not used. Instead, the pharmaceutical company that created the drug will market its use under a brand name.

  2. The **generic name** of a drug is assigned by USAN (the United States Adopted Names Council) to help identify drug action, specifically in the stem of the name. For example, beta blockers all end in *–olol*.

  3. The **brand name**, also known as the trade or proprietary name, is created by the drug company. The FDA must approve all brand names, and the brand name must be distinct from the generic name.

- **Drug interactions** are usually unwanted and can even be harmful. Several types of drug interactions can occur:

  - **Drug-disease interaction**—occurs if the disease alters the absorption, metabolism, or elimination of a drug.

  - **Drug-drug interaction**—occurs when one drug alters the mechanism of another drug.

  - **Drug-dietary supplement interaction**—occurs when the vitamins, minerals, herbs and amino acids in supplements interfere with drug effectiveness.

  - **Drug-laboratory interaction**—occurs when the presence of a drug causes a false positive or negative result.

  - **Drug-nutrient interaction**—occurs when nutrients in food or beverages affect drug effectiveness.

  - **Dosage forms** for medications are generally broken down into solid, liquid, or semisolid. They may also take the form of aerosols, inhalants, and suppositories.

- There are three basic routes of medication administration:

  1. **Oral**—sublingually and buccal

  2. **Parenteral**—intravenous, intradermal, intramuscular, subcutaneous, intra-arterial, intra-articular, and intrathecal

  3. **Topical**—transdermal, ophthalmic, otic, nasal, rectal

- **Side effects** are secondary effects of medications beyond the anticipated or intended effect. The following are some common side effects of medications:

  - Drowsiness

  - Diarrhea/constipation

  - Headache

  - Muscle pain (myalgia)

  - Pain at injection site

  - Sensitivity to sunlight

  - Weight gain

- Harmful or **adverse drug reactions (ADRs)** are unexpected, unintended, undesired, or excessive responses to a drug that cause a variety of negative outcomes.

- **Drug allergies** occur when the immune system responds abnormally to a medication.

- A **drug indication** is the purpose or use of that drug in treating a particular disease. Familiarize yourself with the body systems and disorders for which a drug class is prescribed.

- **Vitamins** are organic substances required for normal body function. **Water-soluble** vitamins are excreted from the kidneys more easily than **fat-soluble vitamins**.

- **Minerals** are necessary for proper functioning of many processes in the body.

- **Supplements** are drugs manufactured to provide nutrients extracted from a plant (herbal) or from synthetic sources to enhance the diet.

- The **stability** of a drug is the length of time the product can retain its chemical, physical and therapeutic properties. Drug stability can also depend on the dosage form of the medication.

- A **therapeutic index** is the dose, or range of doses, of a drug that is most effective without adverse events. Drugs that have a narrow therapeutic index may have requirements for generic substitution, as slight changes in bioequivalence may result in toxicity or ineffectiveness.

- The two main types of incompatibility to be aware of during the compounding process are physical and chemical:

  - **Physical incompatibility** occurs when two or more substances are mixed, and a physical change occurs.

  - A **chemical incompatibility** occurs when a chemical reaction has caused a change in composition, which may include degradation or decomposition of the drug.

- All drugs have specific requirements for storage and handling. Consideration must be given to temperature ranges and sensitivity to light and moisture that will affect medication effectiveness.

PRACTICE QUESTIONS: MEDICATIONS

> **Directions:** Choose the correct answers to the following questions. The answer key and explanations follow the question set.

1. Which of the following is an anticonvulsant?
   A. Cyanocobalamin
   B. Cephalexin
   C. Zolpidem
   D. Carbamazepine

2. The FDA publishes therapeutic equivalence in which reference?
   A. *Trissel's Handbook of Injectable Drugs*
   B. The Orange Book
   C. PDR (*Physicians' Desk Reference*)
   D. Lexicomp

3. The effect antibiotics have on a patient's INR would be considered which type of reaction?
   A. Drug-supplement
   B. Drug-nutrient
   C. Drug-laboratory
   D. Drug-drug (synergism)

4. Which liquid dosage form is used to wash wounds, the bladder, or the eyes?
   A. Enema
   B. Suspension
   C. Irrigation
   D. Elixir

5. While taking which drug should a patient avoid prolonged exposure to sunlight?
   A. Canagliflozin
   B. Fenofibrate
   C. Levothyroxine
   D. Doxycycline

6. Feverfew is used for the treatment and prevention of
   A. menopausal symptoms.
   B. migraine.
   C. anxiety.
   D. arthritis.

7. Which of the following contains a preservative to help prevent the growth of a microbial?
   A. SDV
   B. sublingual tablet
   C. oral antibiotic suspension
   D. MDV

8. Which class of medications often has a narrow therapeutic index (NTI)?
   A. HMG-CoA reductase inhibitors
   B. Anticonvulsant
   C. Antibiotic—Penicillin
   D. ACE inhibitors

9. If two drugs are mixed together and there is a change in color, this would be a
   A. physical incompatibility.
   B. precipitation.
   C. chemical incompatibility.
   D. decomposition.

10. A drug that should be kept refrigerated should be stored at
    A. −25°C to −10°C.
    B. 46°F to 59°F.
    C. −13°F to 14°F.
    D. 2°C to 8°C.

ANSWER KEY AND EXPLANATIONS

1. D	3. C	5. D	7. D	9. A
2. B	4. C	6. B	8. B	10. D

1. **The correct answer is D.** Carbamazepine (Tegretol) is an anticonvulsant. Cyanocobalamin (choice A) is Vitamin B$_{12}$, cephalexin (choice B) is an antibiotic (cephalosporin), and zolpidem (choice C) is a sedative-hypnotic.

2. **The correct answer is B.** The FDA publishes therapeutic equivalence (and generic equivalence) in a reference commonly called the Orange Book. The Orange Book identifies equivalence through therapeutic equivalence (TE) codes. *Trissel's Handbook of Injectable Drugs* (choice A) is a reference for compatibility, stability, storage, and preparation of injectable drugs. The PDR (choice C) is a compilation of prescribing information on prescription drugs. Lexicomp (choice D) is an online reference for drug information.

3. **The correct answer is C.** Antibiotics may alter a patient's INR, and this value is determined during a laboratory test. A drug-supplement interaction (choice A) occurs when a drug interacts with an herbal or dietary supplement. A drug-nutrient interaction (choice B) occurs when nutrients found in food or beverages interact with medications. A drug-drug synergistic interaction (choice D) occurs when two drugs taken together create a greater combined effect than each of the two separately.

4. **The correct answer is C.** An irrigation is fluid used to clean and wash wounds and body cavities, and it can also be used opthalmically. An enema (choice A) is injected into the rectum for bowel cleansing or to deliver medication. A suspension (choice B) is a mixture of particles which do not fully dissolve in liquid. An elixir (choice D) is a liquid that is sweetened and generally contains alcohol.

5. **The correct answer is D.** Tetracycline antibiotics, which include doxycycline and tetracycline, may cause photosensitivity, and patients should be educated to avoid prolonged exposure to sunlight. Canagliflozin (choice A) is an oral hypoglycemic agent and does not cause photosensitivity. Fenofibrate (choice B) is used for hyperlipidemia, and levothyroxine (choice C) is a thyroid hormone; neither cause photosensitivity.

6. **The correct answer is B.** Feverfew is used to treat and prevent migraines. Black cohosh is used for menopausal symptoms (choice A). Kava can be used to treat anxiety (choice C). Glucosamine and chondroitin are used for arthritis (choice D).

7. **The correct answer is D.** An MDV, or multi-dose vial, contains a preservative which allows the vial to be used more than one time. The preservative generally allows an MDV to remain stable for up to 28 days after first puncture. SDVs, or single dose vials (choice A), do not contain a preservative and are used only one time for one person. Sublingual tablets (choice B) are administered under the tongue and, while they may contain dyes or coloring, do not contain a preservative. An oral antibiotic suspension (choice C) is reconstituted with water and has a limited beyond-use date after reconstitution.

8. **The correct answer is B.** Anticonvulsant drugs such as carbamazepine or phenytoin have a narrow therapeutic index, a small window between effective dose and toxicity. HMG-CoA reductase inhibitors, penicillin antibiotics, and ACE inhibitors (choices A, C, and D, respectively) are all prescribed interchangeably with generics and do not have an NTI.

9. **The correct answer is A.** A physical incompatibility results when two or more substances are mixed and a physical change occurs. Precipitation (choice B) occurs when a solid is formed within a solution. A chemical incompatibility (choice C) occurs when a chemical reaction has caused a change in composition. Decomposition (choice D) is a type of chemical incompatibility in which the drug is broken down.

10. **The correct answer is D.** A medication that is kept refrigerated must be stored within the temperature range of 2°C to 8°C or 36°F to 46°F. Choices A and C are incorrect because –25°C to -10°C and –13°F to 14°F are the temperature ranges for frozen medications. Choice B is incorrect because 46°F to 59°F is the range for items to be stored in a cool temperature.

Federal Requirements

OVERVIEW

- **Substance Handling and Disposal**
- **Controlled Substance Prescriptions and DEA Controlled Substance Schedules**
- **Controlled Substances**
- **Restricted Drug Programs and Related Medication Processing**
- **FDA Recall Requirements**
- **Summing It Up**
- **Practice Questions: Federal Requirements**
- **Answer Key and Explanations**

Throughout the years of pharmacy practice, laws, standards, and regulations have been implemented to ensure patient safety and protect pharmacy employees. This chapter highlights safety practices in regard to hazardous drug disposal and handling, and OSHA requirements for safety. It will also discuss federal requirements in terms of controlled substance oversight through the DEA and safety oversight in the recall process through the FDA.

SUBSTANCE HANDLING AND DISPOSAL

Hazardous Drugs

The **Occupational Safety and Health Act of 1970 (OSHA)** established guidelines for safe workplace practices and requirements for employers to provide a safe environment for employees. OSHA established an agency known as the **National Institute for Occupational Safety and Health (NIOSH)**, whose mission is to conduct research and make recommendations regarding employee and workplace safety. One of the evaluations completed by NIOSH is a listing of hazardous drugs. While much of this list is comprised of antineoplastic (chemotherapy) medications, NIOSH defines what makes a drug hazardous, and this list is used to determine the hazardous drugs a pharmacy may have in inventory.

NIOSH defines a drug as hazardous if it displays one or more of the characteristics listed below in human or animal testing:

- Carcinogenicity (causes cancer)
- Teratogenicity or other developmental toxicity (disturbs development of the embryo or fetus)
- Reproductive toxicity (interferes with normal reproduction)
- Organ toxicity at low doses
- Genotoxicity (damages the genetic information of a cell such as DNA or RNA)

Chapter 4

Structure and toxicity profiles of new drugs that mimic existing drugs are determined to be hazardous or not by the above criteria.

OSHA requires a hazard communication program for any facility that stores hazardous drugs. This program must include information regarding labeling of hazardous chemicals, handling and disposal requirements, steps to take in the event of a spill, and an updated safety data sheet (SDS) list. The NIOSH list of hazardous drugs is used to identify what is hazardous in the workplace.

In addition to OSHA regulations, Chapter <800> of the *United States Pharmacopeia (USP)* defines standards for safe handling of hazardous drugs to minimize exposure to both patients and health care workers. In this chapter, standards for handling, storing, administering, transporting, and preparing are defined. USP <800> also uses the NIOSH list to determine if a drug is hazardous.

Handling of Hazardous Substances

Handling requirements for hazardous drugs are contained within a **safety data sheet (SDS)**. An SDS is a document produced by a manufacturer for a chemical or drug deemed hazardous. The SDS contains information about hazardous drug handling, including accidental spills, physical and chemical properties, and disposal information. Below are the sections defined in an SDS. Sections 1–11 are required by OSHA, and sections 12–16 are optional for a manufacturer to provide.

Section	Description of Section
1. Identification	Product Identifier
	Name, address, and phone number of the manufacturer, including emergency contact
	Use and restrictions of the chemical
2. Hazard(s) Identification	Hazard classification and statement
	Pictogram of hazard symbol
	Other hazards not classified
3. Composition and Information on Ingredients	Chemical name, symbol, and any identifiers including mixtures of chemicals
	If a mixture, includes concentration of all ingredients
4. First-Aid Measures	Care that should be given to a person exposed to the chemical
	Instructions based on route of exposure
	Recommendations for immediate medical care and special treatment, if needed
5. Fire-Fighting Measures	Recommendations of fire-extinguishing equipment
	Any hazards which may develop from the chemical during a fire
	Recommendations on special protective equipment or precautions for firefighters

Section	Description of Section
6. Accidental Release Measures	Response to spills, leaks, or accidental release
	Cleanup practices to minimize exposure
	Guidance to distinguish between large and small spills
	Cleanup procedures
	Personal precautions and protective equipment needed
7. Handling and Storage	Precautions for safe handling
	Recommendations for safe storage
8. Exposure Controls and Personal Protection	Appropriate engineering controls, such as laminar flow hood
	Recommendations for personal protective measures to prevent illness or injury from exposure to chemicals
	Any special requirements for PPE, protective clothing, or respirators
9. Physical and Chemical Properties	Physical and chemical properties of the chemical, including odor, pH, and flammability
10. Stability and Reactivity	Reactivity information
	Chemical stability
	Hazardous reaction potential
	Conditions or materials to avoid
11. Toxicological Information	Potential routes of exposure
	Description of effects of exposure, including symptoms
12. Ecological Information	Environmental impact of the chemical
13. Disposal Considerations	Recommendations of appropriate containers for disposal
	Recommendations for appropriate disposal methods
	Guidance on recycling and safe handling practices
14. Transport Information	Guidance on information for shipping and transporting of hazardous chemicals
15. Regulatory Information	Safety, health, and environmental regulations specific to the product that are not indicated anywhere else on the SDS
16. Other Information	Date of latest revision of the SDS

In addition to an SDS, OSHA requires all employers have **personal protection equipment (PPE)** available for employees. For pharmacy technicians, PPE worn in the pharmacy for protection from hazardous drug exposure includes the following:

- Eye shield

- Goggles

- Hair cover

- Beard cover

- Shoe covers (booties)

- Gowns

- Gloves

- Respiratory protection such as face mask

PPE must be worn when compounding and administering hazardous drugs, but should also be worn when receiving, unpacking, or delivering a compounded hazardous drug to the patient. When compounding hazardous drugs, two pairs of chemotherapy gloves must be worn to prevent potential for exposure. In addition, a **closed system transfer device (CSTD)** should be used both to compound and to administer the medication to a patient. CSTDs minimize the risk of hazardous drug exposure to the compounding technician, the nurse or health care worker administering the drug, and the patient.

USP <800> also contains standards for receipt and storage of hazardous drugs. These standards include unpacking hazardous drugs in a designated area of the pharmacy, as well as segregating these drugs when storing in order to prevent additional exposure.

Policies and procedures must also be developed for the prevention of, and response to, a hazardous drug spill. Spill kits must be stocked near the compounding area and where patients may receive hazardous drugs. A spill kit includes shoe covers, gloves, goggles, gown, respiratory mask, chemo spill sign, towels, and sealable bags. If any hazardous drug has come into contact with an employee, the SDS should be referenced for instructions on how to treat the contamination.

Disposal of Non-Hazardous, Hazardous, and Pharmaceutical Waste

Disposal of pharmaceutical waste, both hazardous and non-hazardous, is regulated by the Environmental Protection Agency (EPA) at the federal level, though some state-specific requirements exist. The **Resource and Conservation Recovery Act (RCRA)** established regulations to prevent harm to human health and the environment through the proper management of pharmaceutical waste.

Disposal of waste is summarized in the chart below, which also includes biohazardous waste and sharps information.

Sharps Container	Red Biohazard Container	Yellow Chemotherapy Container	Black Hazardous Waste Container
Needles	Infectious waste	Empty vials used in hazardous drug (HD) compounding	HD bags or vials that are not empty (bulk)
Ampules	Blood products	Empty syringes, needles, or IV tubing used in hazardous drug administration	Gloves, gowns or other PPE that are visibly soiled with HD
Broken glass and other sharps	Material not exposed to chemo but contains blood or bodily fluid	Gowns, gloves, and packaging materials of HD, used when compounding	Specific hazardous drug packaging (P-listed), including warfarin and nicotine patches

Pharmaceutical waste not considered hazardous must be disposed of outside of normal trash disposal, including vials containing drugs that are not on the EPA waste program list. No controlled substances, HD, or sharps should be disposed of with this class. Many sites also segregate aerosols or drugs that may contain a propellant (such as inhalers) due to potential flammability when being incinerated with other pharmaceutical waste.

Some medications may be wasted in a sink drain or a toilet. This includes certain IV bags, such as sodium chloride 0.9% and dextrose, as well as sterile water and lactated ringers. When these bags expire, they are cut open and drained down a sink for disposal, unless state requirements specify otherwise.

CONTROLLED SUBSTANCE PRESCRIPTIONS AND DEA CONTROLLED SUBSTANCE SCHEDULES

The Comprehensive Drug Abuse Prevention and Control Act of 1970, or **Controlled Substance Act (CSA)**, helped pave the way for the Drug Enforcement Administration (DEA) to regulate the manufacturing, distribution, and dispensing of controlled substances. Through the CSA, controlled substances are categorized into five schedules, based on the potential for abuse or dependency and accepted medical use.

The following tables provide a definition and examples of each schedule of controlled substances.

Schedule I (C1)	
Definition	Has no accepted medical use and a high potential for abuse
Examples	• Heroin • LSD (lysergic acid diethylamide) • Marijuana* • Ecstasy 3,4-methylenedioxy-methamphetamine (MDMA)

*Note: In September 2018, the DEA removed some CBD medicines off Schedule I. Specifically, CBD with THC content below 0.1% are now considered Schedule V drugs, as long as they have been approved by the FDA. All other forms of marijuana remain categorized as Schedule I regardless of their approval for recreational and/or medicinal use in various states across the US.

Schedule II (C2)	
Definition	Has accepted medical use, but high potential for abuse, potentially leading to dependence (either physical or psychological)
Examples	• Amphetamine with dextroamphetamine (Adderall) • Fentanyl (Duragesic) • Hydrocodone (Hysingla) • Hydrocodone and acetaminophen (Norco) • Hydromorphone (Dilaudid) • Morphine (MS Contin) • Meperidine (Demerol) • Methylphenidate (Ritalin) • Oxycodone (Oxycontin) • Oxycodone and acetaminophen (Percocet)

Schedule III (C3)	
Definition	Low to moderate potential for abuse, less than Schedule I and Schedule II
Examples	• Anabolic steroids • Testosterone • Codeine with acetaminophen (Tylenol 3) • Ketamine (Ketalar)

Schedule IV (C4)	
Definition	Low potential for abuse and dependence
Examples	• Carisoprodol (Soma) • Clonazepam (Klonopin) • Diazepam (Valium) • Lorazepam (Ativan) • Temazepam (Restoril) • Tramadol (Ultram) • Zolpidem (Ambien)

Schedule V (C5)	
Definition	Little abuse potential (less than Schedule IV) and generally used for antitussive, analgesic, and antidiarrheal purposes
Examples	Codeine with guaifenesin (Robitussin AC) Diphenoxylate and atropine (Lomotil) Pregabalin (Lyrica)

Prescription Requirements

Prescriptions for controlled substances have specific requirements depending on what schedule the drug is. No prescriptions for Schedule I drugs are accepted in a pharmacy, as there is no approved medical use for these medications. All prescriptions for controlled substances must have the following information included:

- Date issued
- Patient's full name and address
- Prescriber's full name and address
- Prescriber's DEA number
- Drug name and strength
- Dosage form
- Quantity prescribed (spelled out—e.g., twenty tablets)
- Directions for use and route of administration
- Number of refills if authorized

A provider must be registered with the DEA to prescribe a controlled substance. A provider may be a physician (either osteopathic or medical doctor), podiatrist, dentist, veterinarian, or mid-level practitioner (physician assistant or nurse practitioner). In order for a prescription to be valid, it must be prescribed for a medical purpose in the field of practice. For example, a dentist could not write a prescription for Norco for back pain.

Below are the credentials for each class of prescribers.

Credential	Profession
MD	Medical Doctor
DO	Doctor of Osteopathy
DPM	Podiatrist
DDS	Dentist (Surgeon)
DMD	Dentist
DVM	Veterinarian
PA	Physician Assistant
CNP	Nurse Practitioner

When a prescriber is registered with the DEA, they will be issued a DEA number, which consists of two letters followed by seven digits. The first letter of the DEA number is either A, B, F, or M, depending on the prescriber's level of practice. The second letter is the first letter of the prescriber's last name. The remaining numbers are a formula designed by the DEA to deter diversion.

Schedule II Prescription Requirements

Schedule II prescriptions may be handwritten or printed from a computer, but must be signed by the prescriber. For electronic systems with DEA certification, they can also be sent electronically through **electronic prescribing of controlled substances (EPCS)**. This process also requires an identification process with the prescriber, to confirm credentials and prescribing eligibility.

Although verbal orders for Schedule II prescriptions are discouraged, in an emergency situation they are permitted. The pharmacy must write out the verbal order as a prescription, and the quantity dispensed must be limited to the amount required for the emergency period. The prescriber must provide the pharmacy with a written prescription for this emergency order within seven days.

Prescriptions for Schedule II medications may not be refilled or transferred. If a pharmacy does not have sufficient quantity to fill the entire prescription, a partial fill may be completed if the remaining quantity can be provided within 72 hours. If the remaining quantity is not available or is not dispensed to the patient within this time frame, a new prescription must be issued.

Schedule III and IV Prescription Requirements

Prescriptions for Schedule III and IV medications may be written, faxed, or called in verbally to a pharmacy. If written or faxed, the order must be signed by the prescriber. These orders may also be sent electronically via EPCS. Refills are permitted for Schedule III and IV prescriptions, though limited to five refills or for six months, whichever occurs first.

A Schedule III, IV, or V prescription may be transferred to another pharmacy once only. However, this rule does exempt pharmacies that share electronic databases, such as those within pharmacy chains. Transfers must meet the following requirements:

- *Void* is written on the original prescription.
- The name, address, and DEA number of the pharmacy where the prescription is transferred must be documented on the back of the original prescription.
- The date of transfer and name of pharmacist accepting the transfer must be recorded.

For a pharmacy receiving a transfer from another pharmacy, the following information must be provided:

- Date of original prescription
- Original number of refills authorized and number of refills remaining
- Date of original dispensing
- Pharmacy name, address, and DEA number from original prescription
- Name of the pharmacist transferring the prescription

Schedule V Prescription Requirements

Prescriptions for Schedule V medications are permitted to be faxed, called in verbally, written, or prescribed through ECPS. These prescriptions may be refilled at the prescriber's discretion, and are not restricted. There are Schedule V medications that may also be purchased without a prescription. Pharmacies are often required to log this information and limit to patients aged 18 years and older.

Schedule	Refills Allowed	Transfer Allowed	Partial Fill Allowed	Verbal or Faxed Orders Allowed
II	No	No	In emergency only; must be within 72 hours	In emergency only; must be within 7 days
III	Up to 5 times within 6 months	One time (unless sharing database)	Yes	Yes
IV	Up to 5 times within 6 months	One time (unless sharing database)	Yes	Yes
V	Up to provider	One time (unless sharing database)	Yes	Yes

CONTROLLED SUBSTANCES

Before a pharmacy can dispense a controlled substance, it must be registered with the DEA. To complete this process, a DEA Form 224 must be submitted, and the pharmacy must renew this DEA license every three years. The DEA certificate of registration must be posted at the pharmacy for inspection.

Ordering Controlled Substances

A controlled substance Schedule I or II must be ordered by a pharmacist using a DEA Form 222 or the controlled substance ordering system (CSOS). The DEA Form 222 is in triplicate—one copy for the purchaser, one copy for the manufacturer or wholesaler, and one copy for the DEA. The pharmacy is responsible for inventorying the DEA 222 forms each month to prevent diversion.

DEA Form 222 has specific requirements for completion. It must list only one item per line, and include the name of the item as well as the number of packages and package size of each item. Only a pharmacist given power of attorney for ordering controlled substances may sign DEA Form 222. The form must be stored in the pharmacy or at an approved off-site location for a minimum of two years.

Schedule III–V controlled substances are permitted to be ordered through standard ordering through the wholesaler or manufacturer, and can be ordered by a pharmacist or a technician.

Receiving Controlled Substances

When a Schedule II controlled substance is received, the invoice must be signed by a pharmacist and stamped with a red C. Each individual line of the invoice must be signed by the pharmacist, with a record of the number of packages received.

Schedule III–V controlled substances can be opened and received by a pharmacist or pharmacy technician. These invoices are not required to be signed by the pharmacist upon receipt.

Invoices of controlled substances must be stored in the pharmacy or an approved off-site location for a minimum of two years.

Storage of Controlled Substances

Schedule II controlled substances must be stored within a vault or safe in the pharmacy. If the medications are stocked at a nursing unit within an **automated dispensing cabinet (ADC)**, the cabinet must be locked, and the medications cannot be stored in an open matrix drawer.

Schedules III–V are permitted to be stored within the secure storage of non-controlled prescription medications. It is up to the pharmacy to determine secure measures for storage of Schedules III–V.

Labeling of Controlled Substances

Manufacturers are required to designate controlled substances by applying a symbol to the label of any scheduled medication. This symbol must be prominently located or large enough for easy identification.

When a controlled substance is dispensed to a patient, the prescription label must contain the standard requirements for all prescription labels, including pharmacy name, address, and phone number; prescriber's name; patient's name; date of fill; and prescription number. In addition, it must also say "Caution: Federal law prohibits the transfer of this drug to any person other than the patient for whom it was prescribed." Pharmacies may often apply additional auxiliary labels to the patient label, which may include "May Cause Drowsiness," "Do Not Drink Alcohol," "May Be Habit Forming," or "Do Not Operate Machinery While On This Medication."

Dispensing of Controlled Substances

Depending on the pharmacy location, there may be specific requirements for pharmacy dispensing on controlled substances. For example, in a hospital, to obtain a controlled substance from an ADC, a nurse requires a witness for verification of dispensing. Some pharmacies require double-counting of all controlled substances before dispensing, including a back-count of the bottle from which the narcotic was dispensed.

Outdated Controlled Substances and Take-Back Programs

When a controlled substance becomes outdated, it must be quarantined from inventory. A pharmacy is responsible for inventorying this outdated inventory monthly to prevent diversion. If a pharmacy destroys controlled substances, a DEA Form 41 must be submitted to the DEA with the name, strength, and quantity of the drug destroyed, as well as a date and method of destruction, including a witness.

Patients may dispose of controlled substances (and other expired or unused medications) through take-back programs, which are designated days sponsored by the DEA. A take-back day allows patients to dispose of any unwanted medications in a safe manner and help patients clean out medication cabinets to prevent inadvertent drug abuse or misuse. In addition to a specified take-back day, many states have year-round or permanent drug disposal programs that utilize safe, onsite disposal boxes or mail-back programs.

Reverse Distribution

If a pharmacy does not have the ability to destroy outdated or damaged controlled substances, this inventory can be transferred to a reverse distributor. A reverse distributor works directly with the DEA and handles the disposal of expired controlled substances. An inventory of all expired items is completed, and then a DEA Form 222 is completed by the reverse distributor to the pharmacy for the controlled substances to be transferred. This DEA Form 222 must also be stored for a minimum of two years. The reverse distributor will then complete its own DEA Form 41 when destroying the controlled substances.

Loss or Theft

If a discovery of a loss or theft is made, the pharmacy must notify the DEA within one business day. The local police department and state board of pharmacy should also be notified, although this is not a federal requirement. A DEA Form 106 must be completed, which can be done online or on paper.

A DEA Form 106 contains the following:

- Name and address of pharmacy
- DEA number
- Date of theft or loss, or when discovered
- If notified, name and phone number of police department
- Type of theft, such as break-in or armed robbery
- Identifying marks, symbols, or price codes used by pharmacy on containers
- Drug name, strength, dosage forms, and package sizes of medications missing

DEA Form Number	Description
41	Destruction of outdated or damaged controlled substances
106	Loss or theft reporting
222	Used for ordering Schedule I or II controlled substances
224	Must be submitted for registration before dispensing controlled substances

Controlled Substance Inventory

A count of all controlled substances must be conducted on the initial inventory and biennially thereafter. The Schedule II inventory must be an accurate, physical count, while the Schedule III–V inventory may be estimated. Inventory records must be kept for a minimum of two years, and the Schedule II inventory must be separated from the Schedule III–V inventory.

RESTRICTED DRUG PROGRAMS AND RELATED MEDICATION PROCESSING

Pseudoephedrine and the Combat Methamphetamine Epidemic Act of 2005 (CMEA)

The **Combat Methamphetamine Epidemic Act of 2005 (CMEA)** set restrictions on the OTC sales of pseudoephedrine, phenylpropanolamine, and ephedrine-containing products. It also defined these drugs as "scheduled listed chemical products."

Specific requirements and restrictions for these products include the following:

- Limit to 3.6 grams daily or 9 grams in a 30-day period

- Required photo ID when purchasing

- Personal records of all purchases are kept for two years

- Customers have limited access—may purchase without prescription but is behind the counter

- Log details of all sales

Pharmacies are responsible for self-certifying annually with the DEA that training and education is completed. Through this certification, the pharmacy is attesting that employees have been educated, records are being maintained, all limits are being enforced, products are not stored outside of the pharmacy, and a logbook is used to track all purchases.

Risk Evaluation and Mitigation Strategies (REMS)

The FDA manages safety of medications through restricted drug programs which require certain medications that may have serious safety concerns to have the risks versus benefits fully evaluated. This is accomplished through **Risk Evaluation and Mitigation Strategies (REMS)**. The purpose of REMS is to prevent, monitor, and manage a risk of medication use by providing education to the patient and health care provider. Without the REMS, the medication would be withdrawn from the market or would not be approved for manufacturing. The manufacturer is responsible for REMS development, after the FDA has identified the need and requirements. REMS can help mitigate adverse events through clinical interventions such as education on specific risks, communication programs, and requiring laboratory testing to monitor effects.

One requirement of REMS may be the development of a **medication (med) guide**. A med guide is a handout given to patients for certain drugs or drug classes. These have additional information describing how to avoid serious adverse effects. The FDA requires a med guide if one of the following conditions exists:

1. Patient labeling could help prevent serious adverse effects.

2. The drug product has serious risk(s) (relative to benefits) of which patients should be made aware because information concerning the risk(s) could affect a patient's decision to use, or continue to use, the product.

3. The drug product is important to patient health, and patient adherence to directions for use is crucial to the drug's effectiveness.

The following drugs and drug classes are some examples of medications required to be dispensed with a med guide:

- Antidepressants

- NSAIDs

- Amiodarone

- Salmeterol

- Salmeterol and fluticasone

- Tamoxifen

Patient package inserts (PPI) contain specific information developed by the manufacturer that is also dispensed with specific classes of products, such as oral contraceptives and estrogen-containing products. Many drug companies may provide the FDA with PPI that is not required but can still be dispensed with products.

Information contained on a PPI includes the following:

- Drug name

- Manufacturer name

- Contraindications and serious associated risks

- Side effects

- Instructions on how to reduce risks

- Date of latest revision of the PPI

REMS may also require direct communication with the manufacturer and health care providers, including pharmacists. This may include interventions, which may reduce serious risk associated with the medication. The FDA may also require that a REMS drug be dispensed or administered in a specific setting only, such as a location that may have access to supplies, personnel, or training for managing a severely adverse event.

Some REMS may even require completion of a certificate or certification in the REMS before being able to dispense the medication. Some of the drugs requiring specific certification programs include clozapine, isotretinoin, and thalidomide.

Clozapine REMS

Clozapine is a drug used to treat schizophrenia. Use of clozapine has been associated with severe neutropenia, which is defined as an absolute neutrophil count (ANC) less than 500 μ/L. Significantly lowered neutrophils can lead to an increased susceptibility to infections.

In order to prescribe, dispense, and take clozapine, REMS must be completed by the provider, pharmacist, and patient. Both inpatient and outpatient pharmacies must be certified in the clozapine REMS program in order to purchase clozapine from a wholesaler. A provider must complete the clozapine REMS program to prescribe clozapine and enroll patients in the REMS program. The prescriber must also report the ANC values to the REMS program to continue providing treatment.

The pharmacy must also become certified in the clozapine REMS program to order and dispense clozapine. The pharmacy must verify that the provider is also enrolled in the program. Before dispensing, the pharmacy validates that the ANC level is appropriate for treatment. Patients must have regular blood tests to confirm ANC level before receiving treatment.

Isotretinoin REMS

Isotretinoin is a drug indicated to treat severe nodular acne. Due to the extremely high risk of birth defects, it must not be used by female patients who are or may become pregnant. Due to the teratogenic effects, isotretinoin is restricted by a REMS program known as iPLEDGE. The goals of this program are to prevent fetal exposure to isotretinoin, and to inform prescribers, pharmacists, and patients about the potential for serious risks.

The iPLEDGE program has specific requirements for providers, patients, and pharmacies. Providers must first be registered with iPLEDGE and may prescribe isotretinoin only to patients who have also registered, and who meet all requirements of the program. The requirements for patients include the following:

- Two negative pregnancy tests prior to the first dose

- Monthly pregnancy tests for female patients to confirm no pregnancy

- Confirmation that two forms of contraceptive are used

- Completion of patient counseling

Once a patient has completed these requirements, isotretinoin can be dispensed. The pharmacy dispensing must also be registered with iPLEDGE. The pharmacy must renew this certification annually, and the wholesaler will only ship the medication if the pharmacy has an active registration. The pharmacy confirms there are no automatic refills on isotretinoin, and prescriptions must be picked up within seven days of the previous negative pregnancy test.

Thalomid REMS®

Thalidomide (Thalomid) is currently indicated for the treatment of multiple myeloma. In the past, it was given to pregnant women as a treatment for morning sickness. As a result, thousands of babies were born with deformed limbs due to its teratogenic effects. Because of this toxicity, thalidomide requires a REMS program for use. The goals of the Thalomid REMS are to prevent the risk of embryo-fetal exposure to thalidomide and to inform prescribers, patients, and pharmacists about the serious risks of use.

The prescriber must first enroll and become certified within the Thalomid REMS program. The prescriber enrolls patients in the REMS program, and must counsel the patient on benefits and risks of thalidomide and provide emergency contraception. Female patients must demonstrate a negative pregnancy test, which the provider will validate. The manufacturer then authorizes the prescriber to write a prescription for thalidomide.

The pharmacy must also certify with the Thalomid REMS program and obtain a confirmation number from the manufacturer before dispensing. Only a pharmacy that is certified can order and dispense thalidomide to registered patients. The pharmacy must also dispense a medication guide with all Thalomid prescriptions.

Opioid Analgesic REMS

A newer REMS established by the FDA was created in response to the treatment of pain. Pain was previously considered a fifth vital sign and was often treated with large doses of opioid analgesics. This practice has created an opioid epidemic and changed the way pain is treated. The goal of the opioid analgesic REMS is to help educate prescribers, pharmacists, and nurses about the treatment and monitoring of patients with pain. These REMS examine the usage of nonpharmacologic treatments and non-opioid analgesics used for pain treatment. This education will provide information about the potential risks using opioids, including inappropriate prescribing, abuse, or misuse.

The opioid analgesic REMS requires manufacturers to provide education for prescribers and pharmacists who may treat pain. Included in this education is information to use when counseling patients on opioid analgesic use.

FDA RECALL REQUIREMENTS

Though FDA-approved medications undergo extensive testing and clinical trials prior to marketing and administration, unexpected issues or problems sometimes occur. When a product is deemed defective or patient use may result in harm, a recall is initiated. A recall ensures either that the drug is removed from supply or the defect is addressed and the drug can be used safely. Manufacturers often initiate a recall voluntarily when discovering an issue. The FDA ultimately oversees the recall process and may instigate a recall for a manufacturer if concerns arise or the manufacturer's process is not sufficient.

There are many products that are regulated by the FDA in the event of a recall, including the following:

- Drugs (both human and animal)
- Medical devices
- Vaccines
- Blood or blood products
- Human tissue transplant
- Cosmetics
- Food for animals
- Products that emit radiation
- Over 75% of the foods eaten in the United States

Recall Classifications

Once a recall has been initiated, it will be classified in one of three classes.

Recall Class	Description	Example
Class I	A product recall involving a product that, if used, could cause serious health problems or death	Test strips reading the wrong INR that causes an increase or decrease in anticoagulation dosing
Class II	A product recall involving a product that might cause a temporary health problem if used, or a slightly serious threat; no immediate danger, but risk of injury is present	Bottles labeled gabapentin 800 mg contain gabapentin 600 mg
Class III	A product recall involving a product that is unlikely to cause any adverse reaction, but violates FDA standards for safety and efficacy	Contamination of a drug with no medical consequences

Pharmacy technicians assist in the recall process by quarantining recalled medications and following the instructions provided by the manufacturer for removal, replacement, or disposal. Pharmacies are not required to notify patients of recalled medications but are required to quarantine recalled medications immediately before they are dispensed to patients.

SUMMING IT UP

- The National Institute for Occupational Safety and Health (NIOSH) defines a drug as **hazardous** if it displays one or more of the following characteristics in human or animal testing:

  - Carcinogenicity (cancer causing)

  - Teratogenicity or other developmental toxicity (disturbance of the embryo or developing fetus)

  - Reproductive toxicity (interferes with normal reproduction)

  - Organ toxicity at low doses

  - Genotoxicity (damages the genetic information of a cell such as DNA or RNA)

- Handling requirements for hazardous drugs are contained within a **safety data sheet (SDS)**, which contains information about hazardous drug handling, including accidental spills, physical and chemical properties, and disposal information.

- Pharmacy technicians must wear **personal protection equipment (PPE)** in the pharmacy for protection from hazardous drug exposure when compounding and administering hazardous drugs and when receiving, unpacking, or delivering a compounded hazardous drug to the patient. In addition, a **closed system transfer device (CSTD)** should be used to both compound and administer the medication to a patient.

- Disposal of pharmaceutical waste, both hazardous and non-hazardous, is regulated by the **Environmental Protection Agency (EPA)** at a federal level, though some state-specific requirements exist.

- The **Drug Enforcement Administration (DEA)** regulates the manufacturing, distribution, and dispensing of controlled substances. **Controlled substances** are categorized into five schedules, based on the potential for abuse or dependency and accepted medical use.

  - **Schedule I (C1):** Has no accepted medical use and a high potential for abuse

  - **Schedule II (C2):** Has accepted medical use, but high potential for abuse, potentially leading to dependence (either physical or psychological)

  - **Schedule III (C3):** Low to moderate potential for abuse, less than Schedule I and Schedule II

  - **Schedule IV (C4):** Low potential for abuse and dependence

  - **Schedule V (C5):** Little abuse potential (less than Schedule IV) and generally used for antitussive, analgesic, and antidiarrheal purposes

- Detailed requirements exist for controlled substance prescriptions based on the schedule of the drug. There is specific information that must be included on all prescriptions, the prescriber must be registered with the DEA, and the prescription must be prescribed for a medical purpose within the prescriber's field of practice.

- The schedule of a controlled substance determines how its prescription may be submitted (signed by the prescriber, called in or faxed in, or sent through EPCS), if (and how many times) it can be refilled, if it is transferable, and if a partial refill is allowed.

- To be allowed to dispense a controlled substance, a pharmacy must be registered with the DEA. DEA guidelines for controlled substance handling procedures include the following:

  - Ordering

  - Receiving

  - Storage

  - Labeling

  - Dispensing

  - Handling outdated inventory (including reverse distribution procedures)

  - Reporting loss or theft

  - Counting inventory

- The purpose of **Risk Evaluation and Mitigation Strategies (REMS)** is to prevent, monitor, and manage risk of medication use by providing education to the patient and health care provider. This information may be communicated through **medication (med) guides** or **patient package inserts (PPIs),** or it may require direct communication with the manufacturer.

- Some REMS may require completion of a certificate or certification in the REMS before a pharmacy may dispense the medication. Some medications requiring such specific training programs include clozapine, isotretinoin, and thalidomide.

- A **recall** is initiated when a product is deemed defective or if patient use may result in harm. A recall ensures either that the drug is removed from supply or that the defect is addressed and the drug can be used safely. Manufacturers often initiate a recall voluntarily, but the FDA ultimately oversees the recall process.

PRACTICE QUESTIONS: FEDERAL REQUIREMENTS

> **Directions:** Choose the correct answers to the following questions. The answer key and explanations follow the question set.

1. Which of the following is established and regulated by OSHA?

   A. Safe handling of hazardous drugs

   B. Safe workplace practices

   C. Scheduling of controlled substances

   D. Notification of recalls

2. A drug that is a carcinogen causes

   A. birth defects.

   B. genetic defects.

   C. reproductive defects.

   D. cancer.

3. Which of the following is a Schedule IV controlled substance?

   A. Lomotil

   B. Lorazepam

   C. Norco

   D. Loratadine

4. A patient has a prescription for Percocet #10 tabs. The pharmacy has 8 tablets in stock, and the patient takes the partial fill. It has been 24 hours since the patient picked up the first fill for this prescription. How much time does the pharmacy have remaining to fill the rest of the prescription before a new order must be obtained?

   A. There is no time remaining; the prescription has expired at 24 hours.

   B. There are no restrictions on obtaining the remainder of the prescription.

   C. 24 more hours

   D. 48 more hours

5. Which DEA form must be completed in the event of a theft?

   A. DEA Form 41

   B. DEA Form 106

   C. DEA Form 222

   D. DEA Form 224

6. Which of the following is a task a pharmacy technician can complete in regard to controlled substances?

   A. Receiving and signing off on Schedule II medications

   B. Registering with the DEA using a DEA Form 222

   C. Ordering Schedule III–V medications

   D. Completing a CSOS order

7. Which of the following medications would require a med guide be dispensed for the patient?

   A. Citalopram

   B. Amoxicillin

   C. Atorvastatin

   D. Lisinopril

8. Which of the following sales would be illegal under the CMEA?

   A. Purchasing 2.4 grams of pseudoephedrine in one day

   B. Purchasing 3.2 grams of pseudoephedrine in 3 days

   C. Purchasing 8 grams of pseudoephedrine in 15 days

   D. Purchasing 12 grams of pseudoephedrine in 21 days

9. A recall initiated because use of the product may cause serious harm or death is

   A. a Class 1 recall.

   B. a Class 2 recall.

   C. a Class 3 recall.

   D. able to be initiated only by the manufacturer.

10. Which of the following drugs is associated with the REMS program iPLEDGE?

    A. Thalidomide

    B. Isotretinoin

    C. Clozapine

    D. Opioid analgesics

ANSWER KEY AND EXPLANATIONS

1. B	3. B	5. B	7. A	9. A
2. D	4. D	6. C	8. D	10. B

1. **The correct answer is B.** OSHA established guidelines for safe workplace practices and requirements for employers to provide a safe environment for employees. Safe handling of hazardous drugs (choice A) is defined in USP <800>. The DEA schedules controlled substances (choice C), and the FDA oversees the recall process (choice D).

2. **The correct answer is D.** A drug that is carcinogenic causes cancer. Drugs that are teratogenic cause birth defects (choice A). Genetic defects (choice B) are caused by drugs that are genotoxic. Exposure to substances with reproductive toxicity may result in reproductive defects (choice C).

3. **The correct answer is B.** Lorazepam is a benzodiazepine, which is a drug class comprised entirely of Schedule IV controlled substances. Lomotil (choice A) is an antidiarrheal agent and is a Schedule V drug. Norco (choice C) is an opioid analgesic and is a Schedule II. Loratadine (choice D) is an antihistamine that is not controlled.

4. **The correct answer is D.** If a pharmacy must do a partial fill on a Schedule II medication, the remainder must be filled within 72 hours.

5. **The correct answer is B.** DEA Form 106 must be completed in the event of a theft or loss of controlled substances. DEA Form 41 (choice A) is used for destruction of controlled substances. DEA Form 222 (choice C) is used to order Schedule II controlled substances, and DEA Form 224 (choice D) is used for initial registration with the DEA.

6. **The correct answer is C.** A pharmacy technician is permitted to order controlled substances that are not Schedule II through regular ordering processes. Choices A, B, and D are incorrect because a pharmacist (not a pharmacy technician) must sign off on all Schedule II medication invoices, register with the DEA for the pharmacy, and complete a CSOS order.

7. **The correct answer is A.** Citalopram is an antidepressant, which is a group of drugs that require a medication guide be dispensed for patient safety. Other classes requiring medication guides would be NSAIDs, such as naproxen or ibuprofen. Amoxicillin (choice B) is an antibiotic, atorvastatin (choice C) is an HMG-CO-A reductase inhibitor, and lisinopril (choice D) is an ACE inhibitor; none of these require medication guides.

8. **The correct answer is D.** Under the CMEA, sales of pseudoephedrine are restricted to fewer than 3.6 grams purchased daily and no more than 9.6 grams per 30 days. Therefore, purchasing 12 grams in 21 days would be illegal. Purchasing 2.4 grams in one day (choice A) would be under the daily maximum. Purchasing 3.2 grams (choice B) and 8 grams (choice C) in more than one day is still under the 30-day limit.

9. **The correct answer is A.** A Class 1 recall is a recall for a product that, if used, could cause serious health problems or death. A Class 2 recall (choice B) is a recall for a product that might cause a temporary health problem if used, or a slightly serious

threat—there is no immediate danger, but risk of injury is present. A Class 3 recall (choice C) is a recall for a product that is unlikely to cause any adverse reaction but violates FDA standards for safety and efficacy. Although a manufacturer may instigate a recall, the FDA ultimately oversees the recall process and may instigate a recall for a manufacturer if concerns arise or the manufacturer's process is not sufficient, so choice D is incorrect.

10. **The correct answer is B.** Due to the teratogenic effects, isotretinoin is restricted by a REMS program known as iPLEDGE. Thalidomide (choice A) requires a REMS program for use to prevent the risk of embryo-fetal exposure. Clozapine REMS (choice C) is associated with management of ANC to prevent patient harm. Opioid analgesics (choice D) utilize a REMS for patient and prescriber safety for pain management.

Chapter 5

Patient Safety and Quality Assurance

OVERVIEW

- High-Alert/High-Risk Medications and Look-Alike/Sound-Alike (LASA) Medications
- Error Prevention Strategies
- Issues Requiring Pharmacist Intervention
- Event Reporting Procedures
- Types of Prescription Errors
- Hygiene and Cleaning Standards
- Summing It Up
- Practice Questions: Patient Safety and Quality Assurance
- Answer Key and Explanations

A **medication error** is any preventable event that may cause patient harm or may lead to inappropriate medication use, including OTC drugs. Pharmacy technicians have a vital role in patient safety and medication error prevention. There are many error prevention strategies and safety measures available to help mitigate potential medication errors. It is important to identify error-prone abbreviations and prescriptions, and to understand how to report any medication-related event. Medication errors can occur at any point in the dispensing process, including during administration. Even having improper hand hygiene can cause a medication error.

HIGH-ALERT/HIGH-RISK MEDICATIONS AND LOOK-ALIKE/SOUND-ALIKE (LASA) MEDICATIONS

High-Alert/High-Risk Medications

The **Institute for Safe Medication Practices (ISMP)** is an organization whose main purpose is to develop tools and research to prevent medication errors. One way to help prevent errors is to identify specific medications and categories of medications which have a heightened risk of harm if used in error. These drugs may or may not have a higher *rate* of medication error incidents, but the outcome of a medication error involving these drugs would pose a higher *risk* to the patient. ISMP publishes a series of lists of high-alert medications that apply to a variety of health care settings.

> **NOTE**
>
> In the tables that follow, certain medications are shown with bolded, upper-case lettering. Remember, **tall man lettering** is an error prevention technique designed to help distinguish between two drugs that may look alike or sound alike.

The following table lists the **"High-Alert Medications in Acute Care Settings"** as defined by the ISMP. Pharmacies can use this list as a tool to develop an internal high-alert/high-risk medications list.

Classes/Categories of Medications
(Abbreviation key: IV—intravenous; IM—intramuscular)
adrenergic agonists, IV (e.g., **EPINEPH**rine, phenylephrine, norepinephrine)
adrenergic antagonists, IV (e.g., propranolol, metoprolol, labetalol)
anesthetic agents, general, inhaled and IV (e.g., propofol, ketamine)
antiarrhythmics, IV (e.g., lidocaine, amiodarone)
antithrombotic agents, including the following: • anticoagulants (e.g., warfarin, low molecular weight heparin, unfractionated heparin) • direct oral anticoagulants and factor Xa inhibitors (e.g., dabigatran, rivaroxaban, apixaban, edoxaban, betrixaban, fondaparinux) • direct thrombin inhibitors (e.g., argatroban, bivalirudin, dabigatran) • glycoprotein IIb/IIIa inhibitors (e.g., eptifibatide) • thrombolytics (e.g., alteplase, reteplase, tenecteplase)
cardioplegic solutions
chemotherapeutic agents, parenteral and oral
dextrose, hypertonic, 20% or greater
dialysis solutions, peritoneal and hemodialysis
epidural and intrathecal medications
inotropic medications, IV (e.g., digoxin, milrinone)
insulin, subcutaneous and IV
liposomal forms of drugs (e.g., liposomal amphotericin B) and conventional counterparts (e.g., amphotericin B desoxycholate)
moderate sedation agents, IV (e.g., dexmedetomidine, midazolam, **LOR**azepam)
moderate and minimal sedation agents, oral, for children (e.g., chloral hydrate, midazolam, ketamine [using the parenteral form])
opioids, including: • IV • oral (including liquid concentrates, immediate- and sustained-released formulations) • transdermal
neuromuscular blocking agents (e.g., succinylcholine, rocuronium, vecuronium)
parenteral nutrition preparations
sodium chloride for injection, hypertonic, greater than 0.9% concentration
sterile water for injection, inhalation and irrigation (excluding pour bottles) in containers of 100 mL or more
sulfonylurea hypoglycemics, oral (e.g., chlorpro**PAMIDE**, glimepiride, gly**BURIDE**, glipi**ZIDE**, **TOLBUT**amide)

Specific Medications
EPINEPHrine, IM, subcutaneous
epoprostenol (e.g., Flolan), IV
insulin U-500 (special emphasis*) (*All forms of insulin, subcutaneous and IV, are considered a class of high-alert medications. Insulin U-500 has been singled out for special emphasis to bring attention to the need for distinct strategies to prevent the types of errors that occur with this concentrated form of insulin.)
magnesium sulfate injection
methotrexate, oral, nononcologic use
nitroprusside sodium for injection
opium tincture
oxytocin, IV
potassium chloride for injection concentrate
potassium phosphates injection
promethazine injection
vasopressin, IV and intraosseous

© Institute for Safe Medication Practices (ISMP) 2018, all rights reserved. Available at **www.ismp.org/recommendations/high-alert-medications-acute-list.**

Look-Alike/Sound-Alike (LASA) Medications

The ISMP also publishes a list of **look-alike/sound-alike (LASA) medications**, known as the **"List of Confused Drug Names."** This list compiles information entered in the medication error reporting tools for ISMP known as **MERP (Medication Errors Reporting Program)** or **VERP (Vaccine Errors Reporting Program)**. Using this data, ISMP has developed tools to help prevent mix-ups in drug names, including using both brand and generic names on prescriptions and labels, indicating the medication purpose on prescriptions, modifying electronic ordering to ensure LASA medications look dissimilar, and managing inventory in a way to help prevent error in product selection.

Below is an example list of some of the look-alike/sound-alike medications on the "List of Confused Drug Names." To view the complete ISMP list, visit the following URL: **www.ismp.org/recommendations/confused-drug-names-list.**

Drug Name	Confused Drug Name
Accupril	Aciphex
Aciphex	Aricept
Activase	TNKase
Actonel	Actos
Adderall	Inderal

Drug Name	Confused Drug Name
Allegra	Viagra
ALPRAZolam	**LOR**azepam
amantadine	amiodarone
am**LODIP**ine	a**MIL**oride
Antivert	Axert
Avandia	Coumadin
Benadryl	benazepril
Benicar	Mevacor
bu**PROP**ion	bus**PIR**one
captopril	carvedilol
car**BAM**azepine	**OX**carbazepine
Cele**XA**	Zy**PREXA**
Cele**XA**	Cele**BREX**
clonaze**PAM**	clo**NID**ine
clonaze**PAM**	**LOR**azepam
Colace	Cozaar
Cozaar	Zocor
Desyrel	**SERO**quel
Diabeta	Zebeta
Diflucan	Diprivan
Doxil	Paxil
e**PHED**rine	**EPINEPH**rine
Flonase	Flovent
FLUoxetine	**DUL**oxetine
glipi**ZIDE**	gly**BURIDE**
Glucotrol	Glycotrol
Huma**LOG**	Humu**LIN**
Huma**LOG**	Novo**LOG**
Humu**LIN**	Novo**LIN**
hydr**ALAZINE**	hydr**OXY**zine
Keflex	Keppra

Drug Name	Confused Drug Name
LaMICtal	LamISIL
lamoTRIgine	levETIRAcetam
lamoTRIgine	levothyroxine
Lanoxin	Naloxone
Levemir	Lovenox
Lopressor	Lyrica
metFORMIN	metroNIDAZOLE
methadone	methylphenidate
metoprolol succinate	metoprolol tartrate
Miralax	Mirapex
morphine	HYDROmorphone
Mucomyst	Mucinex
Neurontin	Motrin
niCARdipine	NIFEdipine
OLANZapine	QUEtiapine
oxyCODONE	HYDROcodone
Paxil	Plavix
prednisoLONE	predniSONE
Pristiq	PriLOSEC
Restoril	RisperDAL
risperiDONE	rOPINIRole
sertraline	cetirizine
sitaGLIPtin	SUMAtriptan
sotalol	Sudafed
traMADol	traZODone
Ultram	Lithium
Wellbutrin SR	Wellbutrin XL
Zantac	ZyrTEC
Zestril	Zetia

ERROR PREVENTION STRATEGIES

Medication errors may be caused by many factors, such as human error, breakdown in procedure, or communication failure. A **near miss** is an event that is caught before reaching the patient. Reporting a near miss is as important as reporting as an actual event because near misses may help identify trends or breakdowns in procedure before reaching the patient. There are several strategies to reduce or prevent medication errors.

Prescription or Medication Order to the Correct Patient

It is an essential role of the pharmacy technician to ensure safe dispensing of a prescription or medication order to the correct patient. Using the "five rights" of medication safety, a pharmacy technician can verify the appropriate information on each patient.

The five rights of medication safety are as follows:

1. The right patient
2. The right drug
3. The right dose
4. The right route
5. The right time

Although some organizations have added "right dosage form" and "right documentation," **The Joint Commission (TJC)**, the accrediting body for hospitals, recognizes the above "five rights" for safe patient medication administration. These may be used in conjunction with other safety measures to prevent medication errors.

Tall Man Lettering

As indicated in the "List of Confused Drug Names," some medications contain uppercase, bolded letters to draw attention to the differences in drug names. This identification method, known as **tall man lettering**, is mostly used in generic pairs, although some name brand drugs may be included. Tall man lettering helps providers distinguish between two drugs when ordering, and it helps pharmacists and technicians verify and fill a prescription or medication order.

The FDA has an approved drug list with requirements for tall man lettering. The ISMP also has a list, though unapproved by the FDA, which is more comprehensive and contains additional medications. This list may be useful in the hospital setting to create an internal policy and procedure and a list to follow for patient safety.

The following table lists examples from the FDA-approved list for drug names with tall man lettering. To view the complete FDA-approved list and the ISMP list of additional drug names with tall man lettering, visit the following URL: **www.ismp.org/recommendations/tall-man-letters-list.**

Drug Name With Tall Man Letters	Confused With
buPROPion	busPIRone
glipiZIDE	glyBURIDE
hydrALAZINE	hydrOXYzine
niCARdipine	NIFEdipine
prednisoLONE	predniSONE
risperiDONE	rOPINIRole

Separating Inventory

There are several types of medications that should be segregated in a pharmacy inventory. The ISMP provides patient safety goals and other standards to outline these methods. Some of the medications requiring separation from inventory are listed below.

Type of Medication	Description
Expired Drugs	Expired drugs must be segregated from in-dated inventory to prevent dispensing the expired drug to patients.
Short-Dated	Medications that will expire soon should have a method for identification (such as a specific color sticker) to identify which medications to use first.
Recalled	Recalled drugs must be quarantined and removed from stock to prevent dispensing.
High-Alert	High-alert medications either must have a method of distinction (such as a high-alert sticker) to identify them or be stored in a segregated area in the pharmacy.
Hazardous Drugs	Drugs deemed hazardous must be stored in a segregated area of the pharmacy to prevent hazardous drug contamination.

In addition, many facilities use **automated dispensing cabinets (ADC)** in nursing units to help secure floor stock and decentralize the pharmacy operations. Inventory in these cabinets must also be separated depending on drug class and type. Hazardous drugs should not be stored in the cabinets (if possible), and drugs that require dilutions, calculations, or complicated preparations should not be stored in the ADC. No bulk bottles should be stored in the ADC; medications should be stocked in unit-dose, unit-of-use, or ready-to-use dosage forms.

Leading and Trailing Zeros

Medication errors may be caused by incorrect dosage when leading zeros are missed and trailing zeros are used. A **leading zero** is the zero that comes before the decimal point, such as 0.5. A **trailing zero** is one that is used after a decimal point, such as 5.0. Leading zeros help clarify dosing and prevent overlooking the decimal point. Alternatively, trailing zeros may cause confusion and potentially could lead to a ten-fold overdose level. If "5.0 mg" is written, it could be misread as "50 mg". The use of trailing zeros and lack of leading zeros is on TJC's official "Do Not Use" List.

Bar Code Usage

Using bar codes in both pharmacy practice and medication administration adds an additional level of safety and error prevention strategy. In a retail pharmacy, bar codes can be used to validate that the correct medication is chosen when the pharmacy technician is filling the prescription. The pharmacist may then use the barcode to verify the prescription for the patient. In a hospital pharmacy, pharmacy technicians can scan medications prior to stocking ADCs, thus adding another check to the process of inventory replenishment.

Nurses and other health care team members administering medications should use **bar code medication administration (BCMA)** procedures. To begin, the patient's wristband is scanned to verify the patient's identity. After patient identity is confirmed, the nurse then views medications due to be administered in the patient's **Medication Administration Record (MAR)**, and—prior to administration—scans the barcode on the manufacturer label or patient label provided by the pharmacy. This barcode should match the scanned medication with the prescribed order to help verify right drug, right dose, right time, and right route. If there is an error in the medication scanned, the nurse will get an alert to notify and investigate prior to administration. While all medications should be scanned prior to being administered, there may be situations which require rapid medication delivery, such as in an emergency code, where a nurse may be unable to scan the medication before administering. Checks are still in place to prevent errors during emergency situations and to ensure the five rights are still confirmed.

Error-Prone Abbreviations

Through pharmacy-reported medication events, the ISMP has identified abbreviations that are prone to errors and should not be used in practice. It is important to be aware of these abbreviations because, although they are identified as error-prone, they may still be seen in practice. When this happens, it is important to confirm the correct abbreviation is used.

ISMP has a list for error-prone abbreviations, as does TJC. The list published by TJC is used as a standard of practice to evaluate safety within a hospital. The expectation is that this list will be included in a policy for use, as well as indicated within the hospital's **electronic medical record (EMR)**. The following list is published by TJC to meet patient safety goals.

Do Not Use	Potential Problem	Use Instead
U, u (unit)	Mistaken for "0" (zero), the number "4" (four) or "cc"	Write "unit"
IU (International Unit)	Mistaken for IV (intravenous) or the number 10 (ten)	Write "International Unit"
Q.D., QD, q.d., qd (daily) Q.O.D., QOD, q.o.d, qod (every other day)	Mistaken for each other Period after the Q mistaken for "I" and the "O" mistaken for "I"	Write "daily" Write "every other day"
Trailing zero (X.0 mg)* Lack of leading zero (.X mg)	Decimal point is missed	Write X mg Write 0.X mg
MS	Can mean morphine sulfate or magnesium sulfate	Write "morphine sulfate"
MSO4 and MgSO4	Confused for one another	Write "magnesium sulfate"

* Exception: A trailing zero may be used only where required to demonstrate the level of precision of the value being reported, such as for laboratory results, imaging studies that report size of lesions, or catheter/tube sizes. It may not be used in medication orders or other medication-related documentation. © Joint Commission Resources: ("*Do Not Use*" *Abbreviation List*). Oakbrook Terrace, IL: Joint Commission on Accreditation of Healthcare Organizations, (2018). Reprinted with permission.

Below are examples of additional recommendations by the ISMP for error-prone abbreviations.

Abbreviation	Intended Meaning	Misinterpretation	Correction
μg	Microgram	Mistaken as "mg"	Use "mcg"
AD, AS, AU	Right ear, left ear, each ear	Mistaken as OD, OS, OU (right eye, left eye, each eye)	Use "right ear," "left ear," or "each ear"
OD, OS, OU	Right eye, left eye, each eye	Mistaken as AD, AS, AU (right ear, left ear, each ear)	Use "right eye," "left eye," or "each eye"
cc	Cubic centimeters	Mistaken as "u" (units)	Use "mL"
D/C	Discharge or discontinue	Premature discontinuation of medications if D/C (intended to mean "discharge") has been misinterpreted as "discontinued" when followed by a list of discharge medications	Use "discharge" and "discontinue"
IN	Intranasal	Mistaken as "IM" or "IV"	Use "intranasal" or "NAS"
HS	Half-strength	Mistaken as bedtime	Use "half-strength" or "bedtime"
q6PM, etc	Every evening at 6 P.M.	Mistaken as every 6 hours	Use "daily at 6 P.M." or "6 P.M. daily"
SC, SQ, sub q	Subcutaneous	SC mistaken as SL (sublingual); SQ mistaken as "5 every;" the "q" in "sub q" has been mistaken as "every" (e.g., a heparin dose ordered "sub q 2 hours before surgery" misunderstood as every 2 hours before surgery)	Use "subcut" or "subcutaneously"
ss	Sliding scale (insulin) or ½ (apothecary)	Mistaken as "55"	Spell out "sliding scale;" use "one-half" or "½"
SSRI	Sliding scale regular insulin	Mistaken as selective-serotonin reuptake inhibitor	Spell out "sliding scale (insulin)"
TIW or tiw	3 times a week	Mistaken as "3 times a day" or "twice in a week"	Use "3 times weekly"

Below are examples of additional recommendations by the ISMP for error-prone drug name abbreviations.

Abbreviation	Intended Meaning	Misinterpretation	Correction
APAP	acetaminophen	Not recognized as acetaminophen	Use complete drug name
HCT	hydrocortisone	Mistaken as hydrochlorothiazide	Use complete drug name
HCTZ	hydrochlorothiazide	Mistaken as hydrocortisone (seen as HCT250 mg)	Use complete drug name

© Institute for Safe Medication Practices (ISMP) 2015, all rights reserved. Available at **www.ismp.org/recommendations/error-prone-abbreviations-list**.

ISSUES REQUIRING PHARMACIST INTERVENTION

Pharmacy technicians help pharmacists with clinical interventions by identifying alerts when filling prescriptions that require pharmacist attention. A pharmacy technician can communicate this information to the pharmacist, but ultimately all clinical judgments must be made by the pharmacist, including OTC recommendations, therapeutic substitutions, and patient counseling. The process of reviewing clinical interventions for potential changes to patient therapy for optimal outcomes is known as drug utilization review.

Drug Utilization Review (DUR)

A **drug utilization review (DUR)** is a review of a prescription to screen for potential drug interactions, allergies, contraindications, appropriate prescribing, and compliance. Though the DUR process was first mandated by the Omnibus Budget Reconciliation Act of 1990 (OBRA 90) for Medicaid prescriptions, many states and most pharmacy prescription software perform a DUR on all patients.

A DUR helps to ensure that patients are taking medications appropriately and in the most effective method to improve their overall health condition. The DUR can be prospective (before the medication is dispensed), or retrospective (after the patient has received the medication). A prospective DUR is completed generally at insurance adjudication or submission, and is electronically reviewed prior to approval.

A DUR identifies potential issues prior to dispensing, such as the following:

- Patient misuse of a medication

- Drug-disease interaction

- Drug-drug interaction

- Inappropriate prescribing, which may be related to duration of treatment or modification in dosing due to age, gender, or pregnancy

- Recommendations for substitutions and therapeutic interchange

- Allergies

Based on the recommendations from the DUR, the pharmacist may choose to proceed with the prescription, contact the provider for a change or clarification, or educate the patient on compliance.

Adverse Drug Event (ADE)

An injury caused by a drug is known as an **adverse drug event (ADE)**. ADEs include adverse drug reactions, overdoses, and harm from the discontinuation of drug therapy. An ADE may also be caused by a medication error. A pharmacy technician may encounter patients with an ADE, and the incident must be communicated to the pharmacist for appropriate reporting and notification of the prescriber.

ADEs are often preventable, and there are often risk factors for patients and drugs that may lead to a higher chance of an ADE. For example, if a patient is taking numerous medications (polypharmacy), some of which may not be clinically necessary, it would pose a risk of an ADE. Age is an additional risk factor, in both the elderly and young patients. Elderly patients are more susceptible to disease-drug interactions and often require adjusted dosing for renal failure. The American Geriatrics Society publishes a list titled the "Updated Beers Criteria for Potentially Inappropriate Medication Use in Older Adults" (known informally as "Beers Criteria" or the "Beers list"), to identify medications and classes of medications which may be inappropriate for geriatric use. This list gives recommendations for prescribing these classes of medication to prevent ADEs in the geriatric population.

Young patients also have a higher risk for an ADE, as dosing is specific (generally to weight) and often more difficult to predict based on age alone. Younger children may also be unable to communicate, which may complicate prescribing.

OTC Recommendation

Patients often self-medicate when using OTC products. Pharmacy technicians may assist a patient in this process by identifying the location of the OTC medications and answering non-clinical questions regarding the OTC medication. If a patient requests a recommendation, the pharmacist must evaluate the symptoms and disease state before recommending a medication. A pharmacy technician is not trained or licensed to make a clinical judgment for a patient or recommend an OTC item. There are additional factors outside of patient symptoms that a pharmacist must consider when recommending a medication, such as disease state and potential for drug interactions.

Therapeutic Substitution

Therapeutic substitution occurs when a medication is substituted for another in the same drug class. This substitution occurs only under the assumption that both drugs are considered to have the same pharmacologic outcome. The purpose of the substitution is to optimize therapy at the lowest cost. If a patient begins treatment on a new medication, and there are other alternatives in the same drug class, the pharmacy may receive a rejected insurance claim with a therapeutic substitution requirement to a less expensive option. For example, if a patient is prescribed Protonix (pantoprazole), the insurance company may reject the claim and suggest Prilosec (omeprazole) as a cheaper starting option. Both medications are proton pump inhibitors used for GERD, so this prescription may undergo substitution. Care must be used when substituting certain drug classes, such as anticonvulsants, hormone therapy, and antidepressants, as patients respond uniquely to each brand, generic and substitute.

Misuse

The **misuse** of a prescription is intentional or unintentional use of a medication outside of the prescribed directions. Misuse also occurs when an individual takes a medication that is not prescribed to him or her, as well as taking a medication for the euphoria or high. Misuse may be due to noncompliance or drug abuse. Prescription drug abuse is a growing problem in the United States and often is driven by the misperception that abusing prescription drugs is safer than using illicit substances.

The most frequently misused drugs include the following:

- Opioid analgesic medications used to treat pain, such as Percocet, Norco, or tramadol

- CNS depressants, such as benzodiazepines used to treat anxiety (alprazolam, diazepam, lorazepam)

- CNS stimulants, such as those used to treat ADHD (Adderall, Ritalin)

Adherence

Medication adherence, also known as **compliance**, is defined as taking a medication as prescribed. There are many reasons patients may become noncompliant to a medication therapy. Patients may be unable to cover the costs of their medication and may take it every other day or cut a tablet in half. The side effects may be significant and lead to adherence issues. Or, the patient may simply forget. As a pharmacy technician, it is important to identify any potential adherence issues with patient therapy and communicate these to the pharmacist. The pharmacy technician's observations could include noticing when a patient refills a medication, if refill requests are consistently too early or too late, or if the patient makes comments regarding the side effects or cost of a drug therapy. Pharmacy technicians interact regularly with patients, and this information is important to gather for the pharmacist to identify adherence issues, possibly before they start. If a patient mentions not being able to remember taking his or her medication or not, recommend a pill box as a daily reminder. Such a suggestion can be helpful for patients as they age and take several medications at different times of day.

Adherence can be calculated as a percentage using the total days' supply for all patient fills divided by the total days in a given period.

$$\text{Adherence \%} = \frac{\text{Total Days' Supply of Patient Fills}}{\text{Total Days}} \times 100$$

For example, if a patient filled a medication for a 30-day supply 3 times in 6 months, the result would be 90 days of total therapy divided by 180 days of total time:

$$\text{30-day supply} \times 3 \text{ refills} = 90 \text{ days' supply of patient fills}$$

$$6 \text{ months} \times 30 \frac{\text{days}}{\text{month}} = 180 \text{ total days}$$

$$\frac{90 \text{ total days' supply}}{180 \text{ total days}} \times 100 = 50\%$$

This patient would have a 50% adherence rate.

Post-Immunization Follow Up

Pharmacists are permitted to give many different vaccinations, depending on state law. Many states allow pharmacists to give all vaccines to patients of all ages. Some states restrict pharmacist administration of pediatric vaccines under a specified age. When a patient requests a vaccination, the pharmacy technician may assist in completing required documentation for the patient, including an informed consent regarding the risks of the vaccine.

Pharmacists must give a copy of the most recent **vaccine information statement (VIS)** with each vaccine given. Patient counseling should be noted when documenting the vaccination in the pharmacy software. A pharmacist should educate patients on potential side effects from the injection and what side effects must be communicated immediately. If an adverse event has occurred, the pharmacist must report it to the **Vaccine Adverse Event Reporting System (VAERS)** for documentation.

Allergies and Drug Interactions

Allergies should be documented each time a patient fills a prescription to verify that no changes have occurred. When a patient reports having no known allergies, it is important to confirm if the patient is referring only to medications or including other substances as well. This distinction is made by the abbreviations NKA and NKDA. If a patient has no known allergies, including all substances and drugs, the proper documentation is NKA. If a patient has no known allergies to medications, the proper documentation is NKDA. This information is an intervention that is caught on a pharmacy's DUR.

NKA	No known allergies
NKDA	No known drug allergies

Drug interactions are also mitigated through the DUR process by the pharmacist. The pharmacy technician should notify the pharmacist for any alerts indicating a potential interaction or allergy.

EVENT REPORTING PROCEDURES

Medication Errors, Adverse Effects, and Near Miss

A medication error may occur at any point in the medication prescribing, filling, dispensing, or administering process, and may or may not cause harm to a patient. Regardless of the damage to a patient, if the medication reached the patient (or, in the case of an error of omission, did *not* reach the patient), it is still considered an error. There are many factors that may lead to a medication error, including poor communication, human error, environmental factors, or lack of training.

As mentioned previously, if a medication error harms a patient, it is considered an **adverse drug event**, or **ADE**. If a medication error occurs, and the patient was not harmed but had the potential of being harmed, it is known as a **potential ADE**. For example, if a patient is prescribed a post-operative dose of IV antibiotics, and the order is missed, it is an error that may not harm the patient but has the potential to harm if the patient develops an infection because of missing the antibiotic dose.

A medication error that is caught before it reaches the patient is known as a **near miss**. Near misses are just as important to monitor, identify, and report as medication errors. These events help identify trends in potential errors, workflow concerns, and prescribing issues.

MedWatch and MERP

Most pharmacies have an internal reporting system used to track medication errors. Reporting errors is very important—not for a punitive response but for identifying trends and potential environmental concerns. There may be an incident report to complete on paper or through an electronic system that collects and stores all of the reporting data.

The FDA has a reporting system for adverse drug and medication safety events known as **MedWatch**. This program provides a voluntary and online reporting tool to report serious adverse events or product quality concerns. It is through this database that the FDA may initiate investigations with manufacturers for potential recalls. Though there is no legal requirement or standard to report adverse events, it is important to notify the FDA when a patient has experienced such an event.

Completing a MedWatch form online is relatively simple, in order to encourage reporting. Below is the information required when reporting through MedWatch:

- Name of drug (and, if medical device, model and serial number)

- Description of the adverse event

- Any concomitant medication use or disease history

- Date event occurred and when medication was started or stopped

- Dosage and directions for use

- The outcome of the event—i.e., did the adverse event stop after the medication was discontinued?

Recall that the ISMP has a reporting database known as the Medication Error Reporting Program, or MERP. While the goals of this program are similar to MedWatch, ISMP cannot initiate recalls or make recommendations to manufacturers. Through MERP, ISMP can identify or learn about underlying causes of errors, distribute this information to organizations for safety guidelines, and provide practice standards for health care institutions and regulatory bodies (such as TJC) for patient safety.

Product Integrity

In addition to errors and adverse events, product integrity issues should also be reported through the appropriate channels (MedWatch and internal reporting). Reportable issues include premature degradation of a medication (assuming it is prior to the drug's expiration date and the medication has been stored properly) and any indication that a drug may be counterfeit. As more patients access medications outside of the United States, the potential for illegitimate medications grows. As a pharmacy technician, it is important to be able to identify when a medication received looks counterfeit. The **Drug Supply Chain Security Act (DSCSA)** was passed in 2013 to help protect patients from counterfeit, stolen, or contaminated substances.

One of the requirements of the DSCSA is that all manufacturers must place a product identifier on each manufactured drug. A wholesaler or pharmacy is not permitted to accept a medication without this product identifier.

The DSCSA requires manufacturers to provide a pedigree (record from production) of a medication to ensure a clean bill of transit from manufacturer to wholesaler for distribution. This pedigree includes the "Three Ts"—transaction history, transaction statement, and transaction information. **Transaction history (TH)** includes transaction information going back to the original manufacturing of the product. **Transaction information (TI)** is the name, strength, dosage form, National Drug Code (NDC), container size, number of containers purchased, lot number, date of purchase and shipment, and business name of address purchasing. The **transaction statement (TS)** is a statement that declares that the manufacturer did not knowingly ship a counterfeit or illegitimate product, has systems in place for proper procedure, and did not knowingly alter any transaction history. A pharmacy must be able to produce this information, either electronically or on paper, for up to six years from purchase date.

Root Cause Analysis (RCA)

If a medication error occurs, it may be necessary to complete a **root cause analysis (RCA)** to help discover potential preventative measures to reduce the possibility of this error occurring again. The purpose of an RCA is to acknowledge human error as a factor for all errors, but to look past this component and identify potential systematic, workflow, or other major issues that contributed to this event. There are several questions to consider when conducting an RCA:

1. What happened?

2. What usually happens?

3. Why did it happen?

4. What can we do to prevent it from happening again?

5. What actions can be measured?

An RCA is completed by a team that was not involved in the actual error itself but is familiar with the area in which it occurred. When conducting an RCA, it is important to differentiate between a root cause and a contributing factor. A **contributing factor** includes situations, circumstances, or workplace conditions that increased the probability an adverse event could occur. Analyzing the contributing factors can help lead to the discovery of the **root cause** and development of a plan for process change and risk mitigation. The process of an RCA begins with data collection and re-creating the event through interviews with all parties involved in the error.

The team completing the RCA must avoid blaming human error as the cause for the adverse event. It is easy to assume that all errors are caused by human factors, and there is no underlying reason behind the mistake. For example, perhaps a nurse programmed a medication incorrectly into the IV pump and the medication infused too quickly, harming the patient. This incident could be identified as a nurse committing a human error when administering the medication. However, upon investigation it is noted that the IV pump did not have the administered drug loaded into the drug library, and the nurse had to override the IV pump for this order. Though the error was human, the underlying factors surrounding this error would be identified through an RCA and can be mitigated to prevent future occurrences of the same or similar events.

TYPES OF PRESCRIPTION ERRORS

Medication and prescription errors can occur for many different reasons. The following are types of prescription errors and tips to help prevent each type.

Prescribing Errors

A **prescribing error** occurs when there is an error in the written order from the prescriber. Prescribing errors can include abnormal dosage or drug strength, insufficient or excessive quantity, wrong route or dosage form, and inappropriate concentration or rate of infusion prescribed. Ordering an incorrect drug could also be considered a prescribing error. This type of error could occur through the prescribing of a medication that is inappropriate based on patient allergies or other contraindications. In addition, a prescribing error could mean a refill was omitted, or that additional directions or clarification of orders are required.

Prescribing errors may also include indication errors. Lack of drug knowledge may cause an error in prescribing due to contraindication or abnormal doses. Indication errors can also result in medication underuse, overuse, or misuse. **Underuse** occurs when a medication that would help the disease state of the patient is inadvertently not prescribed. **Overuse** occurs when a medication is overprescribed, such as prescribing an antibiotic when an infection is not present. **Misuse** occurs when a medication is prescribed that leads to unfavorable outcomes, such as when a contraindication is overlooked and a patient experiences an adverse event.

Prescribing errors are often caused by communication failure either through misinterpretation of handwriting, verbal orders (transcribing), or the use of illegible or confusing abbreviations. Clarifying orders that contain questionable abbreviations can help mitigate risk when filling prescriptions. Additionally, **computerized provider order entry (CPOE)** helps prevent errors by eliminating manual writing of prescriptions. Through an electronic process, providers can pick the dosage that is safe, instead of writing by hand.

Dispensing Errors

A **dispensing error** occurs during the filling and dispensing process to a patient. This error can involve both pharmacy technicians and pharmacists. A dispensing error can result from calculation errors, incorrect patient selection, or inappropriate refills, such as refills dispensed too soon (early refill). Dispensing errors can also include wrong product selection—including wrong strength or dosage form. LASA drugs stored next to each other may account for incorrect drug dispensing. Dispensing an expired medication would also be a dispensing error.

To prevent dispensing errors, it is important to utilize barcode technology to confirm drug product, strength, and dosage form selection. A pharmacy technician must also confirm that the prescription is legible, and not assume any abbreviations, dosages, or information listed. LASA drugs should be stored separately, and inventory should be organized in a way that helps prevent errors from occurring. Tall man lettering should be used for drug distinction.

Administration Errors

An **administration error** occurs when a medication is administered via the wrong route, given to the wrong patient, or at the wrong time. For example, if a patient is to receive a medication as an IV infusion, but is instead administered an IV push, it could lead to a serious adverse event. In addition, medications given at the wrong time can cause harmful effects or exacerbate the disease. For example, patients with Parkinson's disease must take their medication at distinct and specific times. If a dose is delayed (constituting a wrong time error), symptoms may worsen significantly.

An **omission error** is an administration error that occurs when a patient does not receive the medication at all. An omission error may be detected when the patient is due for the next scheduled dose, and it is noticed that the first dose was not administered, or it was omitted.

Administration errors can be prevented through the use of BCMA. Patient's wristbands are scanned to prevent administration to the wrong patient. Scanning the drug prior to dispensing also helps identify if the drug is incorrect, including the route, dose, and dosage form. Utilizing the "five rights" can also help prevent administration errors.

In addition, utilizing IV smart pumps can help prevent errors due to inappropriate infusion rate. IV pumps have drug libraries that include medications and flow rates. If a pump allows for bi-directional compatibility with an EMR, the order from the provider will flow into the pump, and the data from the pump will be documented on the MAR. This functionality also helps to prevent flow rate overrides or parameters that result in inappropriate dosing.

Monitoring Errors

A **monitoring error** may occur if the drug treatment plan for a patient is not evaluated for appropriate prescribing. Monitoring errors can also be indicated by patient response to therapy, as revealed by such measures as reviewing lab results or evaluating signs of drug toxicity. Monitoring errors may often include a lack of response when a patient requires a modification to the prescribed dosing, or conversely, an alteration to the prescribed dosing that is inappropriate based on treatment plan.

Mitigation of monitoring errors may start with sufficient training of nursing staff and caretakers on the negative effects of medication that may indicate toxicity. Providers must also be trained in understanding monitoring methods, such as through vital signs and evaluation of lab results. Continuing education is required by both nursing staff and physicians to maintain their credentials. This education often includes training on current standards or updated guidelines.

When a medication error occurs, it is often helpful to have a category of severity to use in reporting, investigation, and trend identification. The following table lists an adaptation of the medication error categories provided by the Agency for Healthcare Research and Quality (AHRQ).

Category	Description of Error
A	No error occurred, but there was the capacity to cause an error
B	An error occurred, but did not reach the patient (near miss)
C	An error reached the patient, but it is unlikely to cause harm (can include omission error)
D	An error reached the patient and could have required monitoring or interventions to prevent harm
E	An error that may cause temporary harm
F	An error that may cause temporary harm which may require initial or prolonged hospitalization
G	An error that may result in permanent harm
H	An error that may necessitate interventions to sustain life
I	An error that may contribute to or result in death

HYGIENE AND CLEANING STANDARDS

In order to prevent contamination of sterile compounds and potential issues with sterility and stability, the United States Pharmacopeia (USP) outlines standards for sterile compounding in USP Chapter <797>. USP <797> addresses standards for engineering controls (compounding equipment), personnel training and competencies; standard operating procedures and protocols; quality assurance measures, including certification requirements and monitoring, stability and beyond-use dating (BUD); and layout of the facility, including clean room design.

Handwashing, Hand Hygiene, and Personal Protective Equipment (PPE)

Personal Protective Equipment (PPE) and hand hygiene help minimize the introduction of any microbials into the environment when sterile compounding. PPE consists of shoe covers, gowns, gloves, face mask, and hair cover (and beard cover if needed). The process of **garbing** includes the donning of PPE and handwashing steps. Garbing is completed from the dirtiest to cleanest areas of an individual's outside clothing, so shoe covers are donned first in the anteroom, located outside of the buffer (compounding) room. If the pharmacy technician exits the sterile compounding area into the main pharmacy or hospital, new shoe covers should be applied when re-entering. Next, a hair cover and beard cover should be donned, along with a face mask. A face shield is necessary only when preparing hazardous drugs. Following this step, hand hygiene should occur.

Proper handwashing and hand hygiene is an essential part of sterile compounding requirements and a duty of a pharmacy technician for patient safety. The first step of handwashing begins in the anteroom. No jewelry must be worn when compounding. Nail polish and artificial nails are also prohibited, as microbials can gather under artificial nails, and flecks of nail polish can disrupt sterility.

Debris should be removed from under fingernails with a nail pick or cleaner. Hands should be washed with antimicrobial soap up to the elbows with hot water for a minimum of thirty seconds. Hands are dried with lint-free paper towels.

The next step is to don a non-shedding gown over clean scrubs. Gowns may be disposable and are able to be reused during compounding, as long as they are not visibly soiled or torn. Hand hygiene is continued after donning a gown; a surgical alcohol-based hand scrub should be applied and given sufficient time to dry before donning gloves.

Sterile gloves are then applied and disinfected after application using 70% isopropyl alcohol (IPA). This alcohol must dry prior to compounding sterile products. Once compounding is completed, the order of degarbing should be in reverse of the garbing process, starting with sterile glove removal and ending with shoe cover removal.

If compounding hazardous drugs, a chemotherapy gown should be used and sterile chemo gloves applied. Two gloves should always be used when compounding any hazardous drug.

Cleaning Counting Trays and Countertops

Cleaning in a pharmacy is not limited to the sterile compounding area in an institutional setting. Other pharmacies have cleaning requirements as well. All pharmacies must have purified or distilled water available for cleaning and non-sterile compounding. A pharmacy in general is required to be clean and free from clutter for patient safety.

Counting trays are utilized for a majority of patient prescriptions, and often there is a residue that remains following the filling of a medication. Pharmacy technicians must be mindful of cleaning these trays using 70% IPA. It is especially important to clean the counting trays following the dispensing of medications that may cause cross-contamination. **Cross-contamination** occurs when a medication has left a residue that contaminates the next medication being counted, which can be dangerous for patients who have a serious allergy to a medication. If any residue remains following the counting of one of these drugs and contaminates the next patient's prescription, the patient could suffer an allergic reaction.

Countertops should also be cleaned regularly in all pharmacy settings. Using appropriate cleaners for this task is important in order to sanitize and disinfect. Sanitizing reduces the number of microbes present, while disinfecting is designed to kill any microbials.

In an institutional pharmacy, USP <797> recommends a monthly cleaning of walls, ceilings, and any shelves located in the buffer room and anteroom. This cleaning must be documented in a monthly log. Counters in any area within the clean room should be cleaned daily. If a pharmacy is not open 24 hours a day, it is recommended this cleaning occur at the end of the day.

Cleaning Equipment

Understanding how and where to clean depends on the facility standard operating procedures, layout of the compounding area, and which primary engineering control (PEC) is being used for sterile compounding. The International Organization for Standardization (ISO) standards are used to define how clean the air is in a pharmacy room based on levels—the higher the level, the dirtier the air. The ISO level of the air in the anteroom should be no higher than ISO class 8. The buffer room must have a level no higher than ISO class 7, and within the PEC, the ISO level cannot be greater than ISO class 5. Maintaining proper cleaning standards and equipment maintenance helps retain the ISO standard.

Cleaning sterile compounding equipment begins with daily maintenance. If the PEC has been shut off at any time, it should be run for 30 minutes before use. If a horizontal laminar air flow hood is used when compounding non-hazardous drugs, the air is pulled in to the HEPA filter, then blown out horizontally to the worker. Sterile 70% IPA should be used for cleaning and should first start with the bar for hanging IV bags, followed by the sides of the hood using a bottom-to-top motion. Finally, the surface is cleaned using a side-to-side motion, starting at the back of the hood and working to the front in order to avoid damaging the HEPA filter. Cleaning should be done at the beginning of every shift, every thirty minutes (or before every batch if sooner), and if a spill occurs. Each cleaning must be documented in a daily log.

A **compounding aseptic isolator (CAI)**, or glovebox, may also be used to compound non-hazardous products. A CAI is an enclosed hood that ventilates the HEPA-filtered air out through a ventilation system. Pharmacy technicians insert gloved hands into the arms of the CAI to work within an ISO class 5 area. Cleaning is conducted in the same manner with 70% IPA, but also includes the cleaning of the antechamber next to the main compounding chamber.

The HEPA filter for all PECs must be certified every six months. During the certification process, surface samples are taken from the hood surface to verify proper cleaning. Additionally, any pharmacy staff member who may compound must complete competencies to confirm that proper aseptic technique is being followed.

> ## TIP
> The cleaning of PECs is an important task vital to maintaining patient safety. The information presented is intended to provide a general overview; more detailed steps for cleaning PECs can be found at USP <797>. Online sources that provide recommended step-by-step instruction can be found by visiting the following sites:
>
> **www.pppmag.com/documents/ V3N6/CleaningCAIS_P24.pdf**
>
> **www.airscience.com/news/ articlenum/60/how-to-clean- laminar-flow-cabinet**

Other compounding devices include those used for hazardous drug compounding, such as a vertical flow hood or **compounding aseptic containment isolator (CACI)**. A vertical flow hood, or biological safety cabinet, has a vertical flow of air that flows down after HEPA filtration. It is very important not to block the tops of compounding items when using a vertical flow hood. A CACI uses negative pressure to ventilate the air flow out of the ISO class 5 area. Cleaning is conducted in the same manner; however, sporicidal cleaners are recommended to prevent contamination of hazardous drugs.

SUMMING IT UP

- The "five rights" of medication safety are as follows:
  1. The right patient
  2. The right drug
  3. The right dose
  4. The right route
  5. The right time

- A **medication error** is any preventable event that may cause patient harm or may lead to inappropriate medication use. There are many processes and procedures put in place to reduce the occurrences of medication errors.

- The **Institute for Safe Medication Practices (ISMP)** publishes a series of lists of high-alert medications that apply to a variety of health care settings. Pharmacies can use this list as a tool to develop an internal high-alert/high-risk medications list.

- The ISMP also publishes a list of **look-alike/sound-alike (LASA) medications**, to help prevent mix-ups in drug names on prescriptions and labels. The list is compiled from data collected from the ISMP's medication error reporting tools, **MERP (Medication Errors Reporting Program)** or **VERP (Vaccine Errors Reporting Program)**.

- The identification method known as **tall man lettering** helps providers distinguish between two drugs when ordering, and it helps pharmacists and technicians verify and fill a prescription or medication order.

- The following medications should be segregated in a pharmacy inventory: expired, short-dated, recalled, high-alert, and hazardous.

- Using bar codes in both pharmacy practice and medication administration adds an additional level of safety and error-prevention strategy.

- Both the ISMP and **The Joint Commission (TJC)** have created a list of error-prone prescription abbreviations. The list published by TJC is used as a standard of practice to evaluate safety within a hospital.

- Pharmacy technicians help pharmacists with **clinical interventions** by identifying alerts when filling prescriptions that require pharmacist attention. A pharmacy technician can communicate this information to the pharmacist, but ultimately all clinical judgments must be made by the pharmacist.

- The function of a **drug utilization review (DUR)** is to screen for potential drug interactions, allergies, contraindications, appropriate prescribing, and compliance. Based on the DUR recommendations, the pharmacist may choose to proceed with the prescription, contact the provider for a change or clarification, or educate the patient on compliance.

- **Therapeutic substitution** occurs when a medication is substituted for another in the same drug class. This substitution occurs only under the assumption that both drugs are considered to have the same pharmacologic outcome.

- **Medication adherence**, also known as **compliance**, is defined as taking a medication as prescribed.

- An injury caused by a drug is known as an **adverse drug event (ADE)**.

  - ADEs may include adverse drug reactions, overdoses, and harm from the discontinuation of drug therapy.

  - An ADE may also be caused by a medication error as a result of poor communication, human error, environmental factors, or lack of training.

  - If a patient was not harmed by a medication error but had the potential of being harmed, it is known as a **potential ADE**.

  - A medication error that is caught before it reaches the patient is known as a **near miss**.

- The FDA program **MedWatch** provides a voluntary and online reporting tool to report serious adverse events or product quality concerns. Information gathered from this database may initiate investigations with manufacturers for potential recalls.

- The **Drug Supply Chain Security Act (DSCSA)** requires manufacturers to provide a pedigree (record from production) of a medication to ensure a clean bill of transit from manufacturer to wholesaler for distribution.

  - The DSCSA pedigree includes the "Three Ts": **transaction history, transaction statement, and transaction information**.

- If a medication error occurs, it may be necessary to complete a **root cause analysis (RCA)** to help discover potential preventative measures to reduce the possibility of this error occurring again. There are several questions to consider when conducting an RCA:

  1. What happened?

  2. What usually happens?

  3. Why did it happen?

  4. What can we do to prevent it from happening again?

  5. What actions can be measured?

- When conducting an RCA, it is important to differentiate between a root cause and a contributing factor.

- Several types of prescribing errors can occur:

  - A **prescribing error** occurs when there is an error in the written order from the prescriber

  - A **dispensing error** occurs during the filling and dispensing process to a patient.

  - An **administration error** occurs when a medication is administered via the wrong route, given to the wrong patient, or at the wrong time.

  - A **monitoring error** may occur if the drug treatment plan for a patient is not evaluated for appropriate prescribing.

- The hygiene and cleaning standards for sterile compounding is outlined in United States Pharmacopeia (USP) Chapter <797>.

- To ensure patient safety and sterile conditions in the compounding area, specific procedures for handwashing, hand hygiene, and personal protective equipment (PPE) garbing are necessary.

PRACTICE QUESTIONS:
PATIENT SAFETY AND QUALITY ASSURANCE

Directions: Choose the correct answers to the following questions. The answer key and explanations follow the question set.

1. Which of the following is considered a high-risk medication?
   A. Oxytocin IV
   B. Diphenhydramine IM
   C. Lisinopril PO
   D. Pravastatin PO

2. Which of the following is considered one of the patient "five rights"?
   A. Right insurance
   B. Right patient room
   C. Right route
   D. Right prescriber

3. Which type of drug inventory should be quarantined from all others?
   A. Generic drugs
   B. Brand name drugs
   C. Recalled drugs
   D. PO drugs used for diabetes treatment

4. Which medication has the highest potential to be misused?
   A. Warfarin
   B. Glipizide
   C. Venlafaxine
   D. Alprazolam

5. If a patient filled a 30-day supply of a medication two times within a six-month period, what is this patient's adherence rate?
   A. 20%
   B. 33%
   C. 50%
   D. 75%

6. Which of the following would be an example of a near miss?
   A. A patient receives the wrong medication in his prescription bottle.
   B. A pharmacy technician scans the incorrect NDC but changes the drug prior to pharmacist verification.
   C. A nurse administers a medication IM that was intended for IV push.
   D. A patient receives only 30 of a 60-count prescription.

7. CPOE can help prevent which type of prescription error?
   A. Prescribing
   B. Dispensing
   C. Administering
   D. Monitoring

8. An example of an administration error would be

   A. miscalculating a dose.

   B. giving a patient a medication via IV push that is meant to be infused slowly.

   C. missing lab results on a patient to reduce drug therapy.

   D. writing an order for a medication that is inappropriate for the patient's age.

9. For infection control purposes, which of the following should be donned first when garbing?

   A. Sterile gloves

   B. Hair cover

   C. Shoe covers

   D. Gown

10. What should be used to clean counting trays and laminar airflow hoods?

    A. Soap and water

    B. Sterile water

    C. Bleach

    D. 70% IPA

ANSWER KEY AND EXPLANATIONS

1. A	3. C	5. B	7. A	9. C
2. C	4. D	6. B	8. B	10. D

1. **The correct answer is A.** Oxytocin IV is considered a high-risk medication and is on the ISMP list of high-risk/high-alert medications. Diphenhydramine (choice B), lisinopril (choice C), and pravastatin (choice D) are not considered high-risk medications.

2. **The correct answer is C.** The "five rights" of patient care include the right patient, the right drug, the right dose, the right route, and the right time. Although the right insurance (choice A), right patient room (choice B), and right prescriber (choice D) are important for patient safety, these are not used as patient identifiers when administering medications.

3. **The correct answer is C.** Medications that have been recalled must be quarantined from other inventory so as not to be dispensed to a patient. Generic (choice A) and brand name drugs (choice B) are often stored in certain locations based on a pharmacy protocol, but do not need to be separated from stock. All forms of insulin are considered high-alert. Diabetes drugs (choice D) need to be identified as high-alert in some way (with a sticker or stored in a segregated area in the pharmacy). Since they can be dispensed, it is not necessary to quarantine them.

4. **The correct answer is D.** Medications with the highest potential for misuse include opioids, benzodiazepines, and stimulants used to treat ADHD. Alprazolam is a CNS depressant and has a high potential for misuse. Warfarin (choice A) is used as an anticoagulant, glipizide (choice B) is an oral antidiabetic medication, and venlafaxine (choice C) is an antidepressant.

5. **The correct answer is B.** Adherence can be calculated as a percentage using the total days' supply for all patient fills divided by the total days in a given period.

$$\text{Adherence \%} = \frac{\text{Total Days' Supply of Patient Fills}}{\text{Total Days}} \times 100$$

The patient filled a 30-day supply two times:
$$30 \text{ days} \times 2 \text{ months} = 60 \text{ days}$$

$$\frac{60 \text{ Days of Patient Fills}}{180 \text{ Total Days}} = 0.33 \times 100 = 33\%$$

6. **The correct answer is B.** A medication error that is caught before it reaches the patient is known as a near miss. If an error reaches the patient, as in choices A, C, and D, it has the potential to cause an ADE.

7. **The correct answer is A.** CPOE (computerized provider order entry) allows a provider to electronically select an order, which helps eliminate the risk of illegible handwriting, using error-prone abbreviations, or any ambiguity in the written order. CPOE would not specifically help prevent dispensing, administering, or monitoring errors.

8. **The correct answer is B.** An administration error occurs when a medication is administered via the wrong route, given to the wrong patient, or at the wrong time. Miscalculating a dose (choice A) would be a potential dispensing error. Missing lab results (choice C) to monitor therapy would be a monitoring error. Writing an inappropriate order (choice D) would be a prescribing error.

9. **The correct answer is C.** Garbing is completed dirtiest to cleanest, so shoe covers are donned first. A hair cover (choice B) should be donned next, along with a face mask. After appropriate handwashing is completed, a gown (choice D) is donned, followed by a surgical scrub hand hygiene. The last items to be donned are sterile gloves (choice A).

10. **The correct answer is D.** A 70% IPA is used to clean both counting trays (to prevent cross-contamination) as well as laminar airflow hoods. Soap and water (choice A) will not fully disinfect the area, and sterile water (choice B) does not disinfect at all. Bleach (choice C) can be corrosive and harsh on steel if used for hood cleaning, and can be dangerous for counting trays, as any residue remaining can harm patient drugs.

Order Entry and Processing

Chapter 6

OVERVIEW

- **Procedures to Compound Non-Sterile Products**
- **Formulas, Calculations, Ratios, and Proportions**
- **Alligations and Conversions**
- **Sig Codes, Abbreviations, and Medical Terminology**
- **Days' Supply, Quantity, Dose, Concentration, and Dilutions**
- **Equipment/Supplies Required for Drug Administration**
- **Lot Numbers, Expiration Dates, and National Drug Code (NDC) Numbers**
- **Identifying and Returning Dispensable, Non-Dispensable, and Expired Medications and Supplies**
- **Summing It Up**
- **Practice Questions: Order Entry and Processing**
- **Answer Key and Explanations**

Entering prescriptions and medication orders requires knowledge of compounding procedures, calculations, and pharmacy sig codes and abbreviations. Non-sterile compounding is regulated by standards published in USP Chapter <795>. USP <795> outlines requirements for documentation, equipment, and beyond-use dates.

PROCEDURES TO COMPOUND NON-STERILE PRODUCTS

Compounding is the process of combining two or more substances to create a product that is not available as a manufactured drug. A compounded medication is prepared for a specific patient based on a prescribed order. **Non-sterile compounding** refers to compounding products outside of a sterile environment, or a clean room. Compounding medications in a pharmacy allows flexibility in dosing and flavor, and may improve patient compliance.

The compounding process cannot occur without the proper equipment and procedures in place. First, it is necessary to ensure that a clean area is present and proper PPE is worn. Although the full garb used when sterile compounding is not required for non-sterile compounding, gloves must be worn, and a gown, mask, hair cover, and clean scrubs or lab coat are also recommended. These measures are meant to protect employees who may be compounding hazardous substances, or who may be exposed to aerosol particles.

> **TIP**
>
> It is important to know the proper equipment and procedures required for the compounding process. The protective equipment and subsequent procedures are essential for the safe handling of hazardous products.

One of the most commonly used tools in a pharmacy is a **balance**, which is an instrument used to weigh substances. All pharmacies should have a Class A balance, though electronic or digital balances are most commonly used today. With a Class A balance, calibration weights are used to measure the weight of a substance.

Working with the balance involves the use of **weighing papers** or **weigh boats**, which are disposable items that hold the substance to be compounded in place on the balance. The weigh boat or paper is weighed by itself, and then the scale is "zeroed" or cleared so the weight of the boat or paper is not included in the total weight of the measured substance.

Liquid is measured in various types of glassware, including graduated and conical cylinders or beakers. A **graduated cylinder** has a straight side and comes in various sizes for different volume measurements. A **conical cylinder** is cone-shaped and is wider at the top than the bottom. A **beaker** is used not only for measuring liquids but can also be used for mixing or heating. It is also cylindrical, but has a wider base than a graduated cylinder. When measuring volume, it is important to read the measurement at the bottom of the **meniscus,** which is the curved surface of the fluid. Reading the volume at the top of the meniscus would give an inaccurately high interpretation, and less volume would be used than needed. A glass stirring rod may be used when substances need to be dissolved or mixed thoroughly.

To crush or mix powders, a **mortar** and **pestle** is used. The mortar is bowl-shaped, and the pestle is a tool with a rounded end that is useful for crushing and grinding. A mortar and pestle is useful in reducing particle size through pulverization, which is known as **trituration**. Mortar and pestles used for trituration may be glass or porcelain, depending on what type of compound is being produced.

To prepare compounds using gels, pastes, or creams, a spatula can be used for mixing. A **spatula** is a tool with a handle and flat blade on the end. Spatulas are most often stainless steel, although there are also plastic and rubber spatulas. The process of **spatulation** involves the use of a spatula to mix powders, ointments, or other substances together. Spatulation is completed on an **ointment slab**, which is a large slab made of glass that is used for mixing.

Non-sterile compounding often includes the addition of an active ingredient with a vehicle. A **vehicle** is an inactive or inert substance into which an active ingredient can be mixed.

PHARMACEUTICAL COMPOUNDING TERMS & EQUIPMENT	
Term/Equipment	**Definition/Use**
Active Ingredient	The active drug or ingredient in a compound
Beaker	Can be used for liquid measurement, mixing, or heating; cylindrical with a flat edge and a wide base
Calibration Weights	Used to measure the weight of a substance in a Class A balance
Class A Balance	In all pharmacies, used to measure the weight of substances to be compounded
Compounding	The process of combining two or more substances to create a product that is not available as a manufactured drug
Conical Cylinder	A cone-shaped measurement tool that is wider at its top than its bottom; can be glass or plastic
Digital Balance	Often used in place of a Class A balance for weighing compounded substances
Graduated Cylinder	Straight-sided measuring device for liquids that comes in different sizes for volume measurements; can be glass or plastic

Term/Equipment	Definition/Use
Mortar and Pestle	Mortar—a bowl; pestle—tool with rounded end and handle, used to crush tablets or triturate powders
Ointment Slab	Large slab made of glass that is used for mixing
Weigh Boat	A disposable container (usually plastic) that contains the substances for compounding when weighing
Weighing Paper	A disposable paper that holds a small amount of powder or substance when weighing
Vehicle	Inactive or inert substance into which an active ingredient can be mixed

After the proper supplies are identified, it is important to review the **master formula record (MFR)**. This is the "recipe" for the pharmacy, and it helps to standardize practice. It is also a requirement for USP <795> and can be requested upon regulatory survey inspections. The MFR is required to contain the following information:

- Official drug name, strength, and dosage form
- Ingredients, including quantity of each
- Calculations and doses
- Compatibility and stability references
- Equipment needed
- Instructions for mixing
- Labeling information
- Choice of packaging container
- Packaging and storage requirements
- Description of final product
- Quality control procedures

The MFR specifies a procedure to follow for each compound. In addition to the MFR, a compounding record must be completed each time compounding takes place. The compounding record includes the information needed in the MFR, in addition to the following:

- Lot numbers and expiration dates of the components used
- Total quantity compounded
- Name of compounder, approver, and quality control reviewer
- Prescription number
- Assigned beyond-use date (BUD)
- Copy of the patient label
- Any quality control issues

The MFR lists all procedures that may be used in a compounding process. The following table provides examples of specific techniques that may be used in a compounding procedure.

Non-Sterile Compounding Technique	Definition
Geometric Dilution	A way to mix two substances of unequal quantities, starting with the smaller quantity, and mixing in an equal amount of the larger quantity until all of the ingredients have been added
Levigation	Combining a powder with a liquid; for example, mineral oil (for water-soluble bases) and glycerin (for oil-soluble bases)
Spatulation	Using a spatula to mix, usually on an ointment slab
Trituration	Creating smaller particles through crushing, grinding, or pulverizing using a mortar and pestle

Compounding Non-Sterile Products

Ointments

Ointments are semisolid mixtures that contain the highest oil content of the topical dosage forms. Ointments create a barrier on the skin, which provides protection and allows moisture to stay trapped within. **Gels** may also be used for this same purpose, although they have a lower oil content. An ointment is prepared by first selecting the proper base for compounding. Though there are a few different bases used for ointment production, the most common bases are as follows:

- Petrolatum
- Aquaphor
- Polyethylene glycol (PEG)

Once the base has been selected, the ingredient(s) to be mixed are weighed and placed on an ointment slab. Spatulation and geometric dilution are utilized to mix the ingredients. A levigation agent may also be used to smoothen the preparation, or help the solid compound dissolve better. Because an ointment is an oil-based dosage form, mineral oil would be used as a levigating agent. After compounding is complete, the ointment is transferred into an ointment jar for labeling and dispensing.

Mixtures and Emulsions (Creams and Lotions)

An **emulsion** is a mixture of water and oil, which generally do not mix, but are held together with the use of a stabilizing agent. Creams and lotions are examples of emulsions.

In addition to ointments and gels, creams are also used topically for local skin conditions. A **cream** is a semisolid and is a mixture of oil and water. A cream can be a **water-in-oil (w/o) emulsion**, which contains more oil than water, or an **oil-in-water (o/w) emulsion**, which contains more water than oil. A water-in-oil cream has a greasier feel when applied to the skin, whereas the oil-in-water mixture is absorbed quickly and leaves a wet sensation. A base for a cream is chosen based on where the drug is to be applied, as well as the sensitivity of the patient. Creams are thicker than lotions due to higher oil content.

Lotions have the highest water content and are less oily than creams or ointments, which gives lotions a moisturizing property. Lotions are also useful when needing to apply to a large part of the body, as thinner emulsions tend to spread more easily.

To compound creams and lotions, the active ingredient(s) must first be weighed. A mortar and pestle can be used for compounding creams and lotions. Once the powder has been weighed, a wetting or levigation agent is added to give the mixture a creamy consistency. If too much is added, it will be runny, and if too little is added, it will be clumpy. It is important to follow the MFR for these compounds.

Next, the cream or lotion base is added into the mortar and pestle and is mixed thoroughly. A cream should have powder fully dissolved and in solution before adding the base. It is important that the emulsion is mixed thoroughly so that dosing is consistent when the patient uses the cream or lotion.

After thorough mixing, the cream or lotion is placed into a container similar to an ointment jar for labeling and dispensing.

Liquids

There are several types of oral liquid dosage forms previously mentioned that can be compounded:

- Elixirs
- Solutions
- Suspensions
- Syrups

An **elixir** is a sweet, clear solution containing alcohol. The alcohol is used to dissolve the drug into the solution completely. Elixirs are rarely used and should be avoided in children, patients with history of alcohol abuse, and patients on medications that interact with alcohol.

A **solution** is a mixture of liquid and powder in which the powder is completely dissolved. A solution may also be a dilution if additional water or a diluent has been added to the liquid to lower the concentration. Diluting a solution does require an MFR, as the final diluted volume is determined through a prescribed order and pharmacy calculations. Solutions do not require shaking, as the drug is completely dissolved in the liquid.

A **suspension** is a mixture of powder and liquid in which the powder is not fully dissolved. This means suspensions must always be shaken before administering to ensure dispersion of the drug throughout the bottle. Compounding a suspension is completed during the process of reconstitution. Liquid (usually distilled water) is added to a powder in a specified quantity. It is then shaken and labeled for patient use. Compounding of oral suspensions does not require an MFR, as the bottle supplied by the manufacturer gives instructions for reconstitution.

Syrups are a liquid dosage form sweetened with sugar. This is useful in the case of drugs that have an unpleasant taste. Syrups tend to be stickier and are more viscous due to the substances used for sweetening, such as simple syrup or glycerin. Syrups should be avoided by diabetic patients.

Oral liquids may also be flavored for pediatric patients. When a flavoring agent is added, a formula must be followed to determine which flavor should be used with which medication and how much flavoring should be added. Compounding flavoring agents in liquid medications does not change the BUD or stability of the liquid.

Enemas

Another type of solution, though not administered orally, is an **enema**. An enema is used by inserting the liquid into the rectum through the anus, for the purpose of bowel evacuation. An enema is compounded by weighing the desired active ingredient or crushing the tablets of a prescribed strength. For example, if a provider requests a 500 mg antibiotic enema prior to surgery, and the pharmacy stocks 250 mg tablets, two of the 250 mg tablets must be triturated with a mortar and pestle prior to compounding. After weighing or crushing the prescribed active ingredient, the prescribed volume is measured. The active ingredient is mixed thoroughly with the liquid and is then poured into an enema bag for administration.

Although enemas are often compounded in a hospital or institutional pharmacy setting, it is still not necessary to utilize sterile compounding procedures. An enema is safe to compound in a clean non-sterile environment.

Suppositories

Suppositories are solid dosage forms that absorb through the mucous membranes of the body. They are administered into the rectum, vagina, or urethra. Suppositories are compounded using a mold to form the shape needed. There are two types of vehicles used to make suppositories. A plant oil, such as cocoa butter, is used for a base when the suppository should melt at body temperature. These must be stored in the refrigerator to avoid premature dissolving. PEG does not dissolve at body temperature, but within the membranes of the body. When PEG is used as the base, the suppositories do not need to be refrigerated.

Preparing suppositories starts with melting the vehicle chosen into a liquid. The active ingredient is then added and mixed thoroughly. This mixture is poured into the suppository mold, being careful to not overfill. The mold is cooled until it hardens and the finished compound is stored appropriately.

Capsules

Capsules are oral dosage forms that are often useful for patients who have difficulty swallowing tablets. Capsules may be compounded when the prescribed dose is not available in a manufactured product, or if a patient is allergic to a specific additive used in the manufactured version. A capsule is made of a body (or base) and a cap (or head). The sizes of capsules range from 5 (smallest) to 000 (largest).

Capsule Size	Average Amount Contained
5	50 mg
4	150 mg
3	200 mg
2	250 mg
1	300 mg
0	450 mg
00	750 mg
000	1000 mg

Capsules are compounded using a capsule filling machine (when a large number is needed) or through the punch method. The **punch method** is used when the capsule base is selected and the height of the base is equal to the height of the ingredient powder. The compounder can then punch the capsule into the powder to fill the base. This is not always an accurate method, as it is difficult to get the exact same amount of ingredient in each capsule.

TIP

Remember, the larger the capsule size, the smaller amount of medication it contains, because capsules with larger numbers are physically smaller than those with smaller numbers. A capsule size of 3 contains on average 200 mg. A 00 capsule contains approximately 750 mg.

Compounding Beyond-Use Dates

It is important when compounding to determine a BUD for each compounded product. USP <795> has guidelines for calculating BUDs. It is important to note that a calculated BUD cannot extend past an expiration date of any one of the compounded ingredients.

Compounded Product	BUD	Storage Conditions
Non-aqueous oral solid	6 months	Room temperature
Aqueous dosage forms (emulsions, gels, creams, solutions, sprays, or suspensions)	14 days	Refrigerated
Non-aqueous dosage forms (suppositories, ointments)	90 days	Room temperature

FORMULAS, CALCULATIONS, RATIOS, AND PROPORTIONS

Non-sterile compounding, sterile compounding, and filling prescriptions—both inpatient and outpatient—all require a variety of skills and knowledge of pharmacy calculations. The skills needed include knowing the formulas required to complete dosage calculations, conversions, and solving ratios and proportions, as well as understanding abbreviations and terminology encountered when processing prescriptions. This section will review the needed formulas to complete dosage calculations, conversions, and solving ratios and proportions.

> **NOTE**
>
> The Order Entry and Processing knowledge domain constitutes 21.25% of the PTCE. It is important to understand the equipment, procedures, and calculations needed to process and dispense orders.

Formulas (Fractions, Decimals, Percentages)

Fractions

A fraction is a portion of something or a part of a whole. For example, if a patient is prescribed a tablet that is cut in half in order to take a half-tablet daily, this would be considered 1 part out of 2, or $\frac{1}{2}$. The top of the fraction is known as the numerator, and the bottom is known as the denominator. A fraction can be converted into a number by dividing the numerator by the denominator. This often gives a value with a decimal.

$$\frac{1}{2} = 1 \div 2 = 0.5$$

Decimals

Decimals are fractions with denominators that are a power of 10. Numbers to the left of the decimal point are whole numbers greater than one. Values to the right of the decimal point are less than one. As the decimal point moves either to the right or left, the value decreases or increases by a factor of 10.

Thousands	Hundreds	Tens	Ones	Decimal Point	Tenths	Hundredths	Thousandths	Ten thousandths
1000	100	10	1	0	0.1	0.01	0.001	0.0001

To convert a decimal into a fraction, remove the decimal point from the number to get the numerator, and for the denominator, count the number of places to the right of the decimal point.

For example, let's convert 1.5 into a fraction. The numerator equals the number without a decimal point = 15. The denominator equals the places to the right of the decimal = tenths place = 10.

$$1.5 = \frac{15}{10}$$

The rounding of decimals is also important when solving pharmacy calculations. Many calculations are rounded to the tenth place, though some may require rounding to the hundredth and even thousandth place for higher accuracy. To round the value, look at one place past the desired place for rounding (if rounding to the tenths, look at the hundredths; if rounding to the hundredths, look at the thousandths, etc.). If the place one digit past the desired rounding place is equal to 5 or greater, the number should be rounded up. If it is less than 5, the number remains the same.

For example, let's round 6.239 to the hundredths place.

In this number, the 3 is in the hundredths place. That means you will want to look at the number directly following the 3. Because 9 is greater than 5, round the 3 up to 4. The result is 6.24.

Keep in mind that leading zeroes are important for patient safety, and trailing zeroes should not be used.

> **TIP**
>
> Pay careful attention to leading zeros and trailing zeros. When it comes to patient safety, leading zeros should be used. Trailing zeros can lead to confusion and should not be used.

Percentages

A **percent** is one part per hundred. A percentage can be calculated and expressed in three primary ways:

1. As a fraction
2. As a decimal
3. As a ratio

For example, 25% expressed as a percentage equals the following:

- Fraction = $\frac{25}{100}$
- Decimal = 0.25
- Ratio = 25:100

All of these formulas express the same information: 25 parts out of 100.

When calculating percentages, it is first useful to convert the percentage into a fraction, divide the numerator by the denominator, and multiply by 100.

For example, if we start with the fraction $\frac{7}{10}$ determine the percent by dividing 7 by 10:

$$7 \div 10 = 0.7$$

Next, multiply 0.7 by 100 to get the percent value.

$$(0.7)(100) = 70\%$$

It may also be helpful to convert a percentage into a decimal. This is accomplished by dividing the percent value by 100.

$$70\% = \frac{70}{100} = 0.7$$

Calculations (Ratio Proportion and Dimensional Analysis)

Ratios and Proportions

Ratios are used to define the relationship between two quantities. For example, a ratio seen commonly in pharmacy practice is the dose strength in relation to dose volume, such as 5 mg/10 mL. In this case, the ratio is 5:10 and can be written as a fraction, 5 mg/10 mL. This fraction means there are 5 mg in every 10 mL. This is helpful in pharmacy practice when performing calculations. A proportion is an equation of two equal ratios, and is especially useful when determining an unknown quantity if the other three variables are known. For example, using the ratio example from above, if there are 5 mg/10 mL, how many mg are in 20 mL? The ratio proportion method can be used to solve this equation.

To solve a ratio proportion, it is important to first write out the two ratios, keeping the units on the top the same, and the units on the bottom the same. In our example from above, we know there are 5 mg in every 10 mL, but we do not know how many mg are in 20 mL. Keeping the numerator units the same and the denominator units the same is essential to solve this equation.

$$\frac{5 \, mg}{10 \, mL} = \frac{x \, mg}{20 \, mL}$$

Once the proportion is set up, the next step is to solve for x. This is completed through cross multiplying and dividing.

First, we cross multiply:

$$(5)(20) = (x \, mg)(10)$$

Next, to solve for x, divide both sides of the equation by the number multiplied by x. In this equation, that number is 10.

$$\frac{(5)(20)}{10} = \frac{(x \, mg)(10)}{10}$$

Multiply and divide to solve for x. Dividing both sides by 10 will get x by itself.

$$\frac{(5)(20)}{10} = \frac{(x \, mg)(\cancel{10})}{\cancel{10}}$$

$$\frac{100}{10} = x \, mg$$

$$x = 10 \, mg$$

Dimensional Analysis

Dimensional analysis is an additional method used for finding an unknown variable and is useful when numerous conversions must be made. This method utilizes canceling out units, with the result being the fraction or ratio desired. When setting up dimensional analysis equations, it is important to keep the units that are the same on the top and bottom so they can be canceled.

For example, a prescription is written for 15 mg twice daily, and the medication is available in 400 mg/ 150 mL. How many mL is in a single dose for this patient?

Start by determining how many mg are in one dose. The patient is prescribed 15 mg twice daily, so one dose is 15 mg. Set up the dimensional analysis so the units remaining after canceling are the units desired. In this case, we are looking for how many mL in one dose. Cancel like units, then multiply across the top and divide by the product of the denominators:

$$\frac{15 \, mg}{1 \, dose} \times \frac{150 \, mL}{400 \, mg} = \frac{(15)(150 \, mL)}{(1 \, dose)(400)} = \frac{2,250}{400} = \frac{5.625 \, mL}{dose}$$

ALLIGATIONS AND CONVERSIONS

The following section will address the alligation process and measurement system conversions.

Alligations

During non-sterile compounding, it is often useful to mix together the same drug in different strengths, or mix a drug with a diluent or inert ingredient to reduce the concentration. This process can allow for the preparation of a formulation that is different from the strengths of the stocked medications. To calculate these orders, an alligation can be used to determine how many parts are needed from each ingredient. The final product has a strength between the two products use for compounding.

Alligations are solved using a grid or tic-tac-toe board. The percent strength of the higher ingredient is placed in the top left corner, and the lower percent ingredient in the bottom left corner. In the middle square, the desired percentage strength is added.

Higher Strength %		
	Desired Strength %	
Lower Strength %		

The next step is to subtract the percentage desired strength from the higher strength and place this value in the bottom right corner. The same process occurs for the lower strength (ignore the negative value). These values reflect the number of parts needed for the higher strength and lower strengths, respectively.

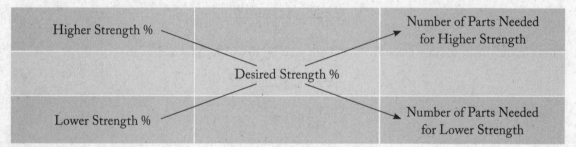

After finding the number of parts needed for both the higher and lower strengths, add these total parts together (add total of right column). This value will give you the total number of parts needed to compound this order.

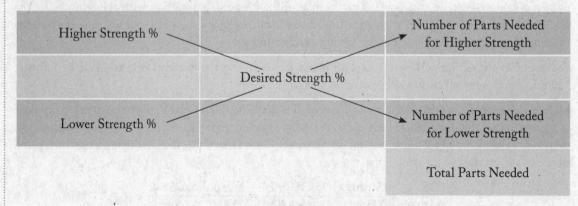

Next, a ratio proportion can be set up to determine the total number of parts needed for each ingredient for the prescribed quantity.

It is important to note that when solving alligations, a diluent such as water, petrolatum, or any other solvent that does not have a strength percentage is entered into the grid as a strength of zero. Alligations can be used to determine the quantity needed for both solids and liquids. If a medication strength is written as a ratio or fraction, it would need to be converted to a percentage prior to completing the alligation.

Example:

Prepare 200 grams of 1.5% hydrocortisone ointment using 2.5% and 1% hydrocortisone base. Determine how many grams of each are required to compound this order.

Solution:

Set up the alligation by putting the higher strength in the top left, lower strength in the bottom left, and desired strength in the middle.

2.5		
	1.5	
1		

Now subtract the difference to find the total parts needed and place this into the top right and bottom right squares.

2.5		**0.5**
	1.5	
1		**1**
		1.5

This means we need 0.5 parts of the 2.5% and 1 part of the 1% hydrocortisone. Adding these together (add the right-hand column): $1 + 0.5 = 1.5$ total parts.

To determine the total grams needed to make the mixture, set up a ratio proportion.

For the 2.5% hydrocortisone:

$$\frac{0.5 \text{ parts}}{1.5 \text{ parts}} = \frac{x \text{ grams}}{200 \text{ grams}}$$

$$(0.5)(200) = (1.5)(x)$$

$$\frac{100}{1.5} = x$$

$$x = 66.7 \text{ grams}$$

66.7 grams of the 2.5% hydrocortisone is needed.

Complete the same process for the 1% hydrocortisone.

For the 1% hydrocortisone:

$$\frac{1\,\text{part}}{1.5\,\text{parts}} = \frac{x\,\text{grams}}{200\,\text{grams}}$$

$$(1)(200) = (1.5)(x)$$

$$\frac{200}{1.5} = x$$

$$x = 133.3\,\text{grams}$$

133.3 grams of the 1% hydrocortisone is needed.

To check your work, add up the total grams needed for each to validate it does equal the total desired.

$$133.3\,\text{grams} + 66.7\,\text{grams} = 200\,\text{grams}$$

Conversions (Measurement Systems)

Metric System

The metric system is the system of measurement most commonly accepted and used around the world, including in the pharmacy practice. There are base units used for length, weight, and volume: meter, gram, and liter. The metric system is based on a factor of 10, and understanding prefixes and conversions within the system is essential to solving dosage calculations.

Below are some common prefixes and the value associated with each when added to a unit.

Prefix	Symbol	Value	Example
Micro–	mc–	One-millionth or 0.000001 × base unit	mcg (microgram)
Milli–	m–	One-thousandth or 0.001 × base unit	mL (milliliter)
Kilo–	k–	One thousand or 1,000 × base unit	kg (kilogram)

Converting between units is important in pharmacy practice and can be completed through three methods.

1. Divide or multiply by 1,000:

   • If converting from a smaller unit to a bigger unit, such as gram to kilogram, divide by 1,000.

   • If converting from a bigger unit to a smaller unit, multiply by 1,000.

2. Move the decimal point:

   • If converting from a smaller unit to a bigger unit, move the decimal point 3 places to the left.

   • If converting from a bigger unit to a smaller unit, move the decimal point 3 places to the right.

3. Set up a ratio proportion:

   Below is a chart showing the conversion for metric units of weight.

Kilogram	Gram	Milligram	Microgram
0.001 kg	1 g	1,000 mg	1,000,000 mcg

Example:

A patient has an order for 350 mg of a medication. How many grams is this?

Solution:

Converting from mg to g is moving from a smaller unit to a bigger unit. Therefore, divide by 1,000 or move the decimal point three places to the left.

Start by setting up a ratio proportion equation:

$$\frac{350\,mg}{x\,g} = \frac{1,000\,mg}{1\,g}$$

Solving for $x = 0.35$ g.

Below is a chart showing the conversion for metric units of volume.

Liter	Milliliter
1 L	1,000 mL

Example:

A patient needs 2.5 L of an oral liquid. How many milliliters is this?

Solution:

Converting from L to mL is converting from a bigger unit to a smaller unit, so to solve, multiply by 1,000 or move the decimal point 3 places to the right. We can start by setting up a ratio proportion equation.

$$\frac{2.5\,L}{x\,mL} = \frac{1\,L}{1,000\,mL}$$

$$x = 2,500\,mL$$

Household System

The **household system** of measurement is still used today to help patients with home dosing. This system is becoming less common due to variances in home dosing supplies. The most frequently encountered household measurements in pharmacy practice are teaspoons and fluid ounces.

Below are the household measurements for volume, and the metric equivalents in mL.

VOLUME		
Household Measurement	**Household Equivalent**	**Metric Equivalent**
1 teaspoon (tsp)	—	5 mL
1 tablespoon (tbsp)	3 tsp	15 mL
1 fluid ounce (fl. oz.)	2 tbsp	30 mL
1 cup (c)	8 fl. oz.	240 mL
1 pint (pt.)	2 c	480 mL
1 quart (qt.)	2 pt.	960 mL
1 gallon (gal.)	4 qt.	3,840 mL

WEIGHT		
Household Measurement	**Household Equivalent**	**Metric Equivalent**
1 ounce (oz.)	—	30 g
1 pound (lb.)	16 oz.	454 g
2.2 pounds (lbs.)	—	1 kg

When converting from lbs. to kg, the ratio proportion method can be used to solve for the unknown value. Another method of conversion to use if the conversion is from lbs. to kg is to divide by 2.2. If the conversion is from kg to lbs., multiply by 2.2. You can remember this by knowing that a person's weight is always higher in pounds than in kilograms.

Example:

A patient weighs 84 lbs. How many kg is this?

Solution:

Use a ratio proportion:

$$\frac{84 \text{ lbs.}}{x \text{ kg}} = \frac{2.2 \text{ lbs.}}{1 \text{ kg}}$$
$$(84)(1) = (x)(2.2)$$
$$84 = 2.2x$$
$$x = 38.2$$

Or, because the conversion is from lbs. to kg, simply divide by 2.2:

$$\frac{84 \text{ lbs.}}{2.2} = 38.2 \text{ kg}$$

It is also helpful to have a quick understanding of mL in fluid ounces, especially when selecting bottle size. Below is a chart of fluid ounce (fl. oz.) conversions and mL volume.

Household Measurement	Volume in mL
1 fl. oz.	30 mL
2 fl. oz.	60 mL
3 fl. oz.	90 mL
4 fl. oz.	120 mL
5 fl. oz.	150 mL
6 fl. oz.	180 mL
8 fl. oz.	240 mL
9 fl. oz.	270 mL
10 fl. oz.	300 mL
11 fl. oz.	330 mL
12 fl. oz.	360 mL

Converting from fl. oz. to mL can be solved by multiplying by 30. If converting from mL to fl. oz., divide by 30. A ratio proportion can always be set up for this conversion as well.

Example:

A patient has a prescription written to dispense 4 fl. oz. How many mL is this?

Solution:

Use a ratio proportion:

$$\frac{4 \text{ fl. oz.}}{x \text{ mL}} = \frac{1 \text{ fl. oz.}}{30 \text{ mL}}$$

$$(4)(30) = (x)(1)$$

$$x = 120 \text{ mL}$$

Or, because the conversion is from fl. oz. to mL, simply multiply by 30:

$$(4 \text{ fl. oz.})(30) = 120 \text{ mL}$$

Apothecary System

The **apothecary system** is an old system of measurement, and some apothecary system units are still encountered in pharmacy practice today. **Grains** are used in measurement of aspirin, phenobarbital, or thyroid medication. **Drams** are often used as measurement for vials used to hold drugs for prescriptions. **Ounces** are also used as a measurement of weight.

The following table details apothecary measurements and metric conversions.

Apothecary Measurement	Metric Equivalent
1 grain	60 mg or 65 mg
1 ounce	30 g

Temperature

In the United States, temperature is often measured using the Fahrenheit scale. On this scale, 32°F is the temperature at which water freezes, and 212°F is the temperature at which water boils. On the Celsius scale, water freezes at 0°C and boils at 100°C. Converting between Fahrenheit and Celsius is important when understanding storage conditions of medications. Pharmacy technicians are responsible for logging temperatures of refrigerators and freezers daily and twice daily if the appliance contains a vaccine.

NOTE

Measurements are an integral part of the pharmacy technician profession. A thorough understanding of the different measurements available, conversion methods, and equivalents is essential.

Below are the equations used to convert between systems.

To convert from Celsius to Fahrenheit: $°F = (1.8 \times °C) + 32$

To convert from Fahrenheit to Celsius: $°C = \frac{(°F - 32)}{1.8}$

Example:

Convert 45°F to Celsius.

Solution:

Using the formula for conversion, enter 45 in for °F:

$$°C = \frac{(45 - 32)}{1.8}$$
$$°C = \frac{(13)}{1.8}$$
$$°C = 7.2°$$

> **TIP**
>
> Understanding how to convert from Fahrenheit and Celsius and vice versa is important for proper medication storage.

SIG CODES, ABBREVIATIONS, AND MEDICAL TERMINOLOGY

In addition to formulas, calculations, and conversions, a pharmacy technician must also be familiar with the language used in prescription writing. This section will review three important components of that language: sig codes, abbreviations, and medical terminology.

Sig Codes

Pharmacy abbreviations used in prescribing are known as **sig codes**. Pharmacy technicians use these for input into the pharmacy software for prescription labels. It is important to be familiar with sig codes for prescription processing.

Below is an example list of pharmacy abbreviations which may be encountered on prescriptions or orders. Prescribers may include periods and often capitalize a number of abbreviations that are listed in lowercase.

Sig Code	Meaning
ac	before meals
ad	right ear
am	morning
amp	ampule
APAP	acetaminophen
as	left ear
ASA	acetylsalicylic acid, aspirin
au	both ears
BID	twice daily
c	with
cap	capsule
cc	cubic centimeter (same as 1 mL)
CMPD	compound
D5W	dextrose 5% in water

Sig Code	Meaning
DAW	dispense as written
DC, D/C	discontinue
DS	double strength
EC	enteric-coated
Elix	elixir
Fl oz	fluid ounce
G, gm	gram
gr	grain
gtt	drop
hr	hour
HS	at bedtime
IM	intramuscular
IV	intravenous
IVP	IV push
IVPB	IV piggyback
mcg	microgram
MDI	metered dose inhaler
mEq	milliequivalent
MOM	milk of magnesia
NPO	nothing by mouth
NS	normal saline 0.9%
od	right eye
oint, ung	ointment
ophth	ophthalmic
os	left eye
ou	both eyes
pc	after meals
PCN	penicillin
pm	evening
PO	by mouth
post	after

Sig Code	Meaning
post op	after surgery
PR	per rectum
PRN	as needed
q	each, every
qd	every day, daily
qhr	every hour
qhs	before bedtime
qid	four times daily
qod	every other day
qs	a sufficient quantity
qwk	every week
s	without
SC, subQ	subcutaneous
sl	sublingual
soln	solution
ss	one-half
STAT	at once, now
subling.	sublingual
supp	suppository
susp	suspension
syr	syrup
tab	tablet
tbsp	tablespoon
tid	three times daily
tsp	teaspoon

Abbreviations

Medical abbreviations are used frequently in pharmacy practice. Below is a list of common medical abbreviations used in prescription writing, and their associated meaning.

Medical Abbreviation	Definition
BM	bowel movement
BP	blood pressure
BPH	benign prostatic hyperplasia
BS	blood sugar
CAD	coronary artery disease
CHF	congestive heart failure
COPD	chronic obstructive pulmonary disorder
GERD	gastroesophageal reflux disease
HA	headache, hyperalimentation
HR	heart rate
HTN	hypertension
MI	myocardial infarction
N & V	nausea and vomiting
RA	rheumatoid arthritis
SOB	shortness of breath
Tx	treatment
Hx	history
Sx	symptoms
URI	upper respiratory tract infection
UTI	urinary tract infection

Roman Numerals

The Roman numeral system is a measuring system that uses letters (either capital or lower case) in place of numbers for value. This numbering system was used in ancient Rome for prescribing pharmaceutical prescriptions, and it is still used today on drug prescriptions to designate quantity or strength and on packaging to designate DEA-assigned schedules for controlled substances.

Below are the Roman numerals used up to 1,000.

Roman Numeral	Number Value
ss	0.5
I or i	1
V or v	5
X or x	10
L or l	50
C or c	100
D or d	500
M or m	1,000

There are several rules to keep in mind when utilizing Roman numerals.

1. The total value of a Roman numeral is the sum of all the numerals, if the values decrease when reading from left to right:

$$XVI = 10 + 5 + 1 = 16$$

2. If a Roman numeral is repeated 3 times, these 3 values should be added (but it cannot be repeated more than 3 times):

$$iii = 3, \text{ but iiii does not equal 4}$$

3. Writing a smaller Roman numeral to the left of a larger numeral requires subtraction:

$$IX = 10 - 1 = 9$$

Example:

A patient's prescription says the following: ii tab po BID × 7d. How many tablets does this patient need for the full prescription?

Solution:

ii = 2

tab = tablets

po = by mouth

BID = twice daily

× 7d = for seven days

The patient will take 2 tablets, twice daily for 7 days = (2)(2)(7) = 28 total tablets needed.

Medical Terminology

Medical terminology is used to understand the meaning of medical words. It consists of one or more root words, prefixes, and suffixes. A prefix is found at the beginning of the word, while a suffix is at the end.

Below are common root words, prefixes, and suffixes for pharmacy practice.

Root Word	Meaning
Aden/o	gland
Cardi/o	heart
Cephal/o	head
Cyst/o	bladder
Derm/o	skin
Erythr/o	red
Gastr/o	stomach
Gyn, Gyn/o	woman
Hemat/o	blood
Hepat/o	liver
Hyster/o	uterus
Leuk/o	white
Neur/o	nerve
Pulm/o	lung
Pyr/o	heat, fever
Ren/o	kidney

Prefix	Meaning
a–, an–	without, not
Brady–	slow
Dys–	bad, difficult
Hemi–	one half
Hyper–	above normal, excessive
Hypo–	below normal, deficient
Intra–	within
Pre–	before
Post–	after
Tachy–	fast

Suffix	Meaning
-algia	pain
-ase	enzyme
-centesis	surgical puncture
-cyte	cell
-ectomy	removal, excision
-emia	blood condition
-gen	production, origin
-gram	recording
-ism	condition, disease
-itis	inflammation
-oma	tumor
-pathy	disease
-scopy	use of an instrument for viewing

Medical terms can be used to build or define words. For example, using the charts above, what would be the medical term for "nerve pain"?

Using the root word for *nerve (neur/o)* and adding the appropriate suffix for *pain (-algia)*, we can combine the word to form *neuralgia*.

DAYS' SUPPLY, QUANTITY, DOSE, CONCENTRATION, AND DILUTIONS

After the pharmacy technician understands the terminology on a prescription, the next step is to provide accurate medications to the patient in terms of number and strength. This section will address the needed skills that contribute to accurately filling the prescription.

Days' Supply and Quantity

Days' supply is defined as how many days the supply of dispensed medication will last. In other words, days' supply is how much medication is needed for a prescription. The correct days' supply is important for safety and clinical appropriateness but is also necessary for proper insurance billing. If the incorrect days' supply is submitted on a claim, the insurance company may reject the claim, or reimbursement could be incorrect.

Pharmacy technicians must be able to calculate days' supply. There are two main ways to calculate, depending on what type of order is being processed.

Total Tablets Needed

Some orders require the calculation of **total tablets needed** to fill the order.

Example:

Take 1 tablet by mouth every 4 to 6 hours for 10 days.

Solution:

- First determine how many tablets will be taken in one day. When calculating this from a range order (e.g., an order in which the dose or dosing interval varies over a prescribed range), assume the patient will take the maximum amount. In this example, every 4 hours = 6×/day.

- Take the total number of tablets taken per day and multiply by the total days of therapy indicated.

This can also be set up as a ratio proportion:

$$\frac{x \text{ tabs}}{10 \text{ days}} = \frac{6 \text{ tabs}}{1 \text{ day}}$$

$$(6)(10) \ = \ 60 \text{ total tablets}$$

How Many Days a Quantity Will Last

Some orders may require the calculation of **how many days a quantity will last**.

Example:

Take 1 tablet by mouth every 4 to 6 hours, dispense 30 tabs.

Solution:

- Again, start with determining how many tablets will be taken in one day. Assume the patient will take the maximum amount = 6×/day.

- Take the total tablets prescribed and divide by the daily dose.

This can also be set up as a ratio proportion:

$$\frac{x \text{ days}}{30 \text{ tabs}} = \frac{1 \text{ day}}{6 \text{ tabs}}$$

$$\frac{30}{6} = 5 \text{ days}$$

In the example above, if the pharmacy had calculated the days' supply using every 6 hours, but the patient ended up taking the medication every 4 hours, the patient would run out of medication before the insurance may allow another refill. This is an example of the importance in days' supply calculations.

Calculating days' supply for insulin is also important so that patients have enough insulin to last them the full time covered by insurance.

Example:

A patient is prescribed Novolog 10 units subQ TID. How long will one vial of insulin last?

Solution:

The first step is to calculate how many units are in one vial. A standard insulin vial is 100 units/mL and contains 10 mL:

$$\frac{x \text{ units}}{10 \text{ mL}} = \frac{100 \text{ units}}{1 \text{ mL}}$$

$$x \text{ units} = (100)(10) = 1,000 \text{ units}$$

There are 1,000 units in one insulin vial.

Next, calculate how many units the patient will be taking daily. The order is written as TID: 10 units × 3 = 30 units daily.

Now divide the total number of units by the daily dose: $\frac{1,000 \text{ units}}{30 \text{ units}} = 33 \text{ days}$.

When calculating days' supply, always round your answer down to the next whole number of days. If a patient has enough for 33.3 days, this should only be considered 33 days.

Dosage Calculations

A **dose** is a specified amount of medication to be taken at a particular time. There are different methods to calculate a dose. Ratio proportion and dimensional analysis can be used to solve dosage calculations. Additionally, some dosing may be weight-based. In these calculations, a medication is usually prescribed in mg of medication per patient weight in kg.

Example:

An order is written for bevacizumab for 5 mg/kg. The patient's weight is 145 pounds. What is the dose for this patient?

Solution:

First, the pounds must be converted into kilograms: $\frac{145 \text{ lbs.}}{2.2} = 65.9 \text{ kg}$

Next, set up a ratio proportion. This problem can also be solved by multiplying the mg dose by the total kg weight of the patient.

$$\frac{x \text{ mg}}{65.9 \text{ kg}} = \frac{5 \text{ mg}}{1 \text{ kg}}$$

Solve for x.

$$x = (65.9)(5) = 329.5 \text{ mg}$$

Body Surface Area (BSA)

Some medications have precise dosing based on **body surface area (BSA)**. Examples of BSA dosing include some pediatric chemotherapy orders. A **nomogram** is a chart used to determine a patient's BSA based on weight and height. BSA is measured in m^2.

Example:

A patient has an order for a medication for 30 mg/m^2. The patient has a BSA of 1.8 m^2. What is the total dose for this patient in mg?

Solution:

This order can be found by simply multiplying the patient's BSA by the mg dose prescribed. It can also be calculated using ratio proportion.

$$\frac{x\,mg}{1.8\,m^2} = \frac{30\,mg}{1\,m^2}$$

$$(30\,mg)(1.8\,m^2) = 54\,mg$$

Other Dosage Strengths

Milliequivalents (mEq)

A **milliequivalent** is a unit of measure used for many electrolytes. In pharmacy practice, mEq are often encountered when calculating doses for total parenteral nutrition (TPN). Electrolytes include potassium (K), sodium (Na), calcium (Ca), and magnesium (Mg).

Example:

A patient has an order for 75 mEq of potassium. The pharmacy has a stock of potassium in 40 mEq/2 mL. How many mL are needed for this dose?

Solution:

Set up a ratio proportion:

$$\frac{x\,mL}{75\,mEq} = \frac{2\,mL}{40\,mEq}$$

Solve for x:

$$x\,mL = \frac{(2)(75)}{40}$$

$$x = 3.75\,mL$$

Units

Units, also known as **International Units**, are another form of measurement used for specific medications such as insulin, heparin, and some vitamin dosing.

Example:

A patient needs a bolus dose of heparin 5,000 units. Heparin is available as a 1,000 unit/1 mL vial. How many mL is needed for this bolus?

Solution:

Set up a ratio proportion:

$$\frac{x\,\text{mL}}{5,000\,\text{units}} = \frac{1\,\text{mL}}{1,000\,\text{units}}$$

Solve for x:

$$x\,\text{mL} = \frac{(5,000)(1)}{1,000}$$
$$x = 5\,\text{mL}$$

Percent Concentration (w/v, w/w, v/v)

Percent concentrations are defined as **weight/volume (w/v)**, **weight/weight (w/w)**, or **volume/volume (v/v)**.

Percent weight/volume (w/v) describes the number of grams in 100 mL of a solution. For example, if the pharmacy stocks a 5% solution, there are 5 grams of active ingredient in 100 mL of solution. The total volume can then be used to determine how much active ingredient is in the solution.

Example:

A pharmacy stocks D5W in 500 mL bags. How much dextrose is in one 500 mL bag?

Solution:

Dextrose w/v = 5%, or 5 grams Dextrose in 100 mL water

To determine the total amount of dextrose in 500 mL, set up a ratio proportion:

$$\frac{x\,\text{grams}}{500\,\text{mL}} = \frac{5\,\text{grams}}{100\,\text{mL}}$$

Dimensional analysis can also be used:

$$\frac{5\,\text{grams}}{100\,\text{mL}} \,\bigg|\, 500\,\text{mL}$$

Percent weight/weight (w/w) describes the number of grams of a medication in 100 grams of a total compound. For example, if you have a 2.5% hydrocortisone, that means there are 2.5 grams of hydrocortisone in 100 grams.

Example:

How many grams of hydrocortisone are in a 2% hydrocortisone cream with a package size of 15 grams?

Solution:

Start with setting up a ratio proportion:

$$\frac{x \text{ grams}}{15 \text{ grams}} = \frac{2 \text{ grams}}{100 \text{ grams}}$$

Dimensional analysis can also be used:

$$\frac{2 \text{ grams}}{100 \text{ grams}} \left| \frac{15 \text{ grams}}{} \right.$$

Both methods are solved by $\frac{(2)(15)}{100} = 0.3 \text{ grams}$

Percent volume/volume (v/v) describes how many mL are in 100 mL of solution. Thus, a 70% IPA contains 70 mL alcohol in 100 mL total solution.

Example:

A pharmacy technician adds a 5 mL of a stock solution into 250 mL of water. What is the percent v/v?

Solution:

Start with setting up a ratio proportion. In this problem, we do not know the percent concentration, but we can find it based on the new stock formula and using 100 mL as our base percentage.

$$\frac{x \text{ mL}}{100 \text{ mL}} = \frac{5 \text{ mL}}{250 \text{ mL}}$$

Dimensional analysis can also be used:

$$\frac{5 \text{ mL}}{250 \text{ mL}} \left| \frac{100 \text{ mL}}{} \right.$$

Both methods are solved by $\frac{(5)(100)}{250} = 2 \text{ mL} = \frac{2 \text{ mL}}{100 \text{ mL}} = 2\%$

Dilutions

It is often necessary to dilute stock solutions to a lesser concentration or greater volume. Calculating dilutions can be accomplished using the formula:

$$(C_1)(V_1) = (C_2)(V_2)$$

C_1 = Concentration of stock

V_1 = Volume or weight of stock

C_2 = Final concentration of desired product

V_2 = Final volume or weight of desired product

Example:

An order is written for 500 mL of a 12% solution. You have a 20% solution in stock. How much stock solution and how much diluent are needed to compound this order?

Solution:

$C_1 = 20$

$V_1 = x$

$C_2 = 12$

$V_2 = 500$

Solve for x:

$$(20)(x) = (12)(500)$$

$$x = \frac{(12)(500)}{20} = 300$$

$$x = 300 \text{ mL of stock solution is needed.}$$

This question also asks for quantity of diluent needed with the stock solution. This can be found by taking the final volume and subtracting the stock volume calculated:

$$500 \text{ mL} - 300 \text{ mL} = 200 \text{ mL}$$

200 mL diluent is added to 300 mL stock solution to get a final volume of 500 mL.

EQUIPMENT/SUPPLIES REQUIRED FOR DRUG ADMINISTRATION

When dispensing prescriptions to patients, it is important for the pharmacy technician to select the appropriate packaging for medication administration. In a community pharmacy setting, unless a waiver has been signed, all packaging should be child resistant, unless the medication falls into the "Exempt" list from the Poison Prevention Packaging Act. Some examples of exemptions include sublingual nitroglycerin, oral contraceptives, and hormone replacement therapy.

Package Size

In a retail pharmacy, oral solids, such as tablets and capsules, are packaged in amber vials after counting. Although not all medications are light-sensitive, this amber bottle prevents potential degradation from light. The sizes of amber prescription bottles are still measured in drams, with the smallest size being a 6 dram bottle all the way up to a 60 dram bottle. When selecting the appropriate size for patients, use the counting tray spout to pour the counted medication into the bottle. It is important to use the size that is the closest fit to the quantity dispensed without overfilling the bottle.

For liquid medications, amber bottles are also used, but these are measured in fluid ounces. When selecting an appropriate size bottle for liquid medications, once again, it is important to not overfill the bottle. Understanding the conversion of fluid ounces to mL is important when selecting the appropriate bottle size. For instance, if a patient has an order written for 150 mL, the 4 fl. oz. bottle would be too small, and the 6 fl. oz. bottle should be used (depending on what size the pharmacy has in stock).

Below is a chart of the most commonly sized bottles for fluid. Many pharmacies will choose to stock just the 4, 8, and 10 fl. oz. bottles. Some pharmacies may stock 0.5 fl. oz. (15 mL) with a dropper for pediatric doses.

Bottle Size	Volume in mL
1 fl. oz.	30 mL
2 fl. oz.	60 mL
3 fl. oz.	90 mL
4 fl. oz.	120 mL
6 fl. oz.	180 mL
8 fl. oz.	240 mL
10 fl. oz.	300 mL
12 fl. oz.	360 mL

Unit Dose

In a hospital or institutional pharmacy setting, medications are dispensed as **unit dose**, which is a drug packaged for a single administration. For example, when unit dose medications are purchased from a wholesaler, they are often packaged in a box of 100 in 10 sheets of 10 tablets. These tablets can be torn off for individual use.

The FDA requires each unit dose label to contain the following information:

- Drug name and strength
- Expiration date
- Lot number
- Name of manufacturer
- Special dosage form characteristics, such as ER tablet, enteric-coated, chewable
- Bar code

The FDA recommends, but does not require, the following information:

- NDC number
- Special storage requirements
- Special administration requirements (such as shake before use)

Unit dose formulations can be solid oral dosage forms such as tablets, capsules, or chewable or ODT tablets. There are also liquid unit dose cups that are packaged in a one-dose form for solutions or suspensions.

Unit dose offers significant benefits to the hospital workflow, including efficiency in medication preparation, since a dispensing cabinet can be stocked with unit dose medications. It also helps reduce medication errors, as unit dose medications can be scanned by a nurse prior to administration. Additionally, unit dose drugs help reduce wastage and improve cost effectiveness. If a patient does not use a medication, it can be returned to the pharmacy for dispensing to another patient as long as the packaging is intact.

Repackaging Medications

Hospitals may find that unit dose medications are more expensive than bulk bottles. This is generally true for most medications, but dispensing medications in unit dose form is a requirement for institutional facilities. To help alleviate some of this cost, pharmacies may repackage medications from bulk bottles into unit dose packaging. Repackaged medications must also be labeled appropriately and include a barcode for scanning at administration.

It is important to recognize the definition of **repackaging**. The FDA accepts repackaging as removal of a finished drug from the original manufacturer container to be placed into a different packaging without any manipulation of the drug. This means if a medication is reconstituted, diluted, or modified in any way, it is not considered repackaged.

Pharmacies must document all repackaged medications. A log is kept, which includes the information required on the label as well as the quantity repacked. The log also requires the signatures of the technician performing the repacking and the pharmacist verifying accuracy.

Repackaged medication labels must include in the following:

- Name and address of pharmacy repacking
- Drug name, strength, and dosage form
- Lot number (pharmacy batch number)
- Manufacturer name and lot number
- Date of repackaging
- BUD

The BUD calculated depends on the formulation and the expiration date of the drug being repackaged.

Formulation	BUD
Non-liquid formulations	6 months, or expiration date of drug if sooner
Water-containing oral formulations	14 days, or expiration date of drug if sooner
Water-containing topical/dermal formulations	30 days, or expiration date of drug if sooner

Unit-of-Use

Unit dose and repackaging are forms of medication that allow for a one-dose administration to a patient. A unit-of-use package is a medication that is labeled in the original manufacturer container that contains a sufficient quantity for a course of therapy. For example, oral contraceptives are packaged in a 28-day supply. It is not beneficial to remove these tablets from the packaging and put them into a bottle. Other medications may be manufactured in 30-, 60-, or 90-count bottles that are appropriate to dosing method. For example, a medication taken once daily may be packaged in a 30-count bottle to provide sufficient quantity for a one-month supply. The same would be true for a medication taken twice daily that is packaged in a 60-count bottle, or taken three times daily in a 90-count bottle. When preparing these medications as a prescription, a label can simply be applied directly to the manufacturer packaging.

Diabetic Supplies

For patients with diabetes, understanding what supplies are needed for what purpose can be challenging. It is important for pharmacy technicians to understand the supplies used to manage diabetes. Many of these supplies are are classified as **durable medical equipment (DME)**. DME can also include crutches, canes, walkers, or other medical devices used to assist patients.

Because diabetic patients must be able to continuously monitor blood glucose levels, a **glucometer** can be recommended for at-home testing. A glucometer uses a specific type of test strip to identify blood glucose levels. A patient uses a **lancet** to pierce the skin and draw blood. Blood is placed onto the test strip, which is then inserted into the glucometer for reading. The test strips are disposed of after each use and cannot be reused. It is important to have the test strips that work specifically with the type of glucometer a patient may own, as each glucometer uses its own specific test strip.

If patients are required to self-administer insulin daily, they will also need insulin syringes for administration. These syringes come in sizes based on the prescribed dosage. This includes 0.3 mL, 0.5 mL, and 1 mL syringes. Insulin syringes are specialized, as they are measured in both mL and insulin units for accurate dosing.

Newer formulations of insulin are often administered using **insulin pens**. Insulin pens contain a prefilled insulin cartridge and a dial for measuring dosage. Insulin pens offer a convenient and accurate method of dosing, but are more expensive than insulin in vials. Insulin pens require needles for administration, known as pen needles. These needles are smaller in size and are less painful than insulin syringes.

Respiratory DME

In addition to diabetic supplies, some patients may require DME for respiratory purposes. Younger patients needing respiratory medication administration may require a spacer or nebulizer.

A **spacer** is a chamber that is attached to an MDI. When the inhaler is puffed, the aerosolized medication can stay in the spacer, rather than escape into the air if not administered properly. The patient can then breathe in the medication directly from the spacer for higher drug absorption. Spacers are available in various sizes, depending on the age of the patient.

Nebulizers are machines that take the solution from a respiratory nebule (such as albuterol) and turn it into a mist for inhalation. Nebulizers are often used on pediatric patients and are hooked to a tube and mask that the patient wears. The nebule is opened and poured into the nebulizer. The machine will then aerosolize the liquid through tubing until a mist is formed. The patient can then breathe in the mist and receive the drug administered through the mask at the end of the tubing.

Oral and Injectable Syringes

Syringes are used for medication administration for both oral and sterile medications. There are three basic types of syringes:

1. Hypodermic
2. Insulin
3. Tuberculin

Hypodermic syringes are typically plastic syringes that range in size from 3 mL to 60 mL. These syringes can be used for oral administration. An **oral syringe** is used for liquid medications most commonly administered to pediatric patients. Oral syringes are used without a needle for administration, but allow for more precise dosing than other medication cups or household measurement tools. When a syringe is used to draw up a medication for oral administration, a syringe cap is attached to the tip to prevent medication from being removed from the syringe.

Medications such as IM or IV Push can be administered through a hypodermic syringe and needle. A needle can also be attached to a hypodermic syringe for sterile compounding. When compounding sterile products, syringe selection is important to provide the most accurate dosing. Selecting the smallest syringe that can hold the desired volume is the best way to provide precise dosing.

Insulin syringes are used for diabetic patients for insulin administration. These syringes are 1 mL or less and are measured in both mL and units for insulin dosing. Insulin syringes typically range from 30 units (0.3 mL) up to 100 units (1 mL).

Tuberculin syringes are small syringes that hold up to 1 mL and are used for intradermal administration of a purified protein derivative (PPD). This injection helps indicate if a person has tuberculosis (TB). PPD skin tests are generally completed on employees working in a healthcare field prior to beginning work.

Regardless of the type, all syringes are composed of the same parts. Most syringes are made of plastic or polyvinyl chloride (PVC). The main components include the plunger, barrel, and seal. The **plunger** is used to draw medication into or eject medication out of the syringe. The **barrel** is the tube that holds the medication and has calibration lines for measurement, which vary depending on the size of the syringe. The black rubber **seal** is located at the end of the plunger within the syringe, and its top (the side closest to the tip of the syringe) is the appropriate place for reading measurements. The **tip** of the syringe is a point of attachment for needles or oral syringe caps.

Syringe tips are typically one of two types: slip-tip or luer lock. A **slip-tip syringe** is used less frequently in practice, as this type of syringe holds a needle in place through friction only. Needles may slip off if not pushed on tightly. **Luer lock syringes** are used more frequently. A luer lock is a threading mechanism that allows a needle to screw into place for a secure fit.

Needles

Needles are used for medication administration of injectable doses and for sterile compounding. There are three main components of a needle: hub, shaft, and bevel. The **hub** is the bottom part of the needle that secures into the syringe. The **shaft** is the long stem of the needle, which is sharpened at one end to create a point at the needle tip. The **bevel** of the needle is the opening at the end.

The size of a needle is determined by the length and gauge. The length of the needle is measured from the spot of joining between the hub and the shaft to the tip of the needle. Lengths of needles range from $\frac{3}{8}$ inch up to 6 inches. The **gauge** of a needle is a measurement of the diameter, or how wide the needle is. The **gauge** value has an inverse relationship with the size of the needle, meaning the larger the gauge value, the thinner the needle. Needle gauges range from 6 G to 32 G, although the most commonly used range is from 15 G to 25 G. The diameter of the needle increases as the gauge number decreases. Small gauge (i.e., wider) needles are used for more viscous solutions, as the wider needles can withdraw and administer these solutions more easily. Larger gauge (i.e., thinner) needles are used to minimize pain for patients during injection.

Below is a description of needle gauges and an example of use for each.

Needle Gauge (G)	Examples of Use
15 G	Withdrawing and administering viscous solutions
16 G	IV infusion—large volumes
20–22 G	IM injection IV infusion
22–24 G	IV infusion for continuous infusions being infused slowly
25 G	Subcutaneous injections
26–28 G	Intradermal injections
30–32 G	Ultra-fine pen needles for diabetic use

LOT NUMBERS, EXPIRATION DATES, AND NATIONAL DRUG CODE (NDC) NUMBERS

Lot Numbers

A **lot number** is a number assigned by a manufacturer to a specific batch of drugs produced. Lot numbers are used for tracking purposes by both the manufacturer and the purchaser.

Manufacturers utilize lot numbers for quality control and to identify ingredients for supply chain security. In addition, if a manufacturer must initiate a recall, the lot number is used to identify which batch of medication must be recalled. Pharmacies can then use this information to pull the specific lot number from inventory and quarantine the supply. Lot numbers are indicated on the drug packaging, often next to the expiration date.

Expiration Dates

The **expiration date** of the drug is the last date the manufacturer can guarantee stability, purity, and quality of the medication produced. If a manufacturer indicates an expiration date as just a month and year, the drug is good through the last day of the month. For example, if the expiration date listed is 4/2025, this drug expires on 4/30/25. Pharmacy technicians have an important role in removing medications from shelves, dispensing cabinets, and floor stock prior to expiration.

National Drug Code (NDC) Numbers

The Drug Listing Act of 1972 required the use of a **National Drug Code (NDC)** number for all drugs produced by FDA-registered manufacturers. An NDC number is a unique number comprised of 10 digits, grouped into 3 segments. Both prescription and OTC medications must have an NDC number, and the FDA maintains a database of all NDCs. Although a 10-digit NDC is required, 11 digits are utilized for billing purposes. This means if a manufacturer publishes a 10-digit NDC, the pharmacy will add a 0 in a specified location.

The first set of numbers in an NDC represents the **Labeler,** which is the manufacturer, repackager, or distributor. The labeler code consists of 5 numbers, but if a manufacturer uses the 10-digit NDC format, a 0 is added at the beginning of the first 5. For example, if a labeler code is 1234, the pharmacy will utilize the 5-digit format of 01234. The FDA assigns the labeler code to manufacturers.

The second and middle set of numbers of the NDC identifies the product. This is known as the **product code**, and it specifies the drug strength and dosage form of the drug. For example, if the same manufacturer produces both tablets and capsules of the same drug, the product code would be different, even though the drug is the same, because the dosage forms are different. The product code consists of 4 numbers, or it can be 3 numbers in a 10-digit format. If the product code is 567, a 0 would be added to the beginning for pharmacy billing purposes and would be entered as 0567.

The third set of numbers designates the **package size**. This number describes the package size and type. The package code is 1 or 2 digits long. If the manufacturer utilizes a 10-digit NDC, the package code may be 1 digit, and a 0 is added before that digit. For example, if the package size is 8, the pharmacy would utilize 08. When comparing NDCs, if a manufacturer produces the same drug and dosage form both in a pack of 10 units and also a pack of 100 units, the NDCs will be the same until the last 1 or 2 digits.

The **NDC number** is found on the drug packaging with the lot number and expiration date, as well as on the drug container itself, such as a vial or bottle. There is a barcode on all drug containers, and the NDC number is embedded into the barcode so that when it is scanned, the correct drug can be identified during medication administration. Below is an example of an NDC number in the 5-4-2 (11-digit) format.

$$\underbrace{12345}_{\text{Labeler Code}} - \underbrace{6789}_{\text{Product Code}} - \underbrace{10}_{\text{Package Code}}$$

It is often helpful to know when and where to add a 0 when converting from a 10-digit NDC to the 11-digit, 5-4-2, format. Below are examples of 10-digit NDCs and the 11-digit conversion for each.

10-Digit Format	Example of NDC Format	11-Digit Conversion
4-4-2	2222-2222-22	02222-2222-22
5-3-2	33333-333-33	33333-0333-33
5-4-1	44444-4444-4	44444-4444-04

IDENTIFYING AND RETURNING DISPENSABLE, NON-DISPENSABLE, AND EXPIRED MEDICATIONS AND SUPPLIES

Managing inventory in the pharmacy involves continuous monitoring of expired drugs, utilizing reverse distributors for expired medication credit and prescriptions that can be returned either to stock or to the wholesaler. While all pharmacies maintain individual procedures for these processes, it is important to know that if a prescription is given to a patient and leaves the pharmacy, it cannot be returned or re-dispensed. Once a drug is no longer in the possession of the pharmacy, it cannot be verified for purity, quality, or strength.

Credit Return

Vigilant inventory management is important for managing pharmacy drug expenditures and total inventory cost. If a medication was ordered in error, or if a medication was ordered in excess and is still on the shelf (a slow mover), it may be eligible for return to the wholesaler. This scenario could occur if a patient was receiving a specialized medication and then has the therapy discontinued. The drug being returned cannot have been opened or damaged, and generally is restricted in expiration dating, meaning if the drug expires soon (short-dated), the wholesaler may not take the return. Prior approval is given from the wholesaler for the returned medications, which is defined in the wholesaler return procedure. Wholesalers may also indicate if specific medications are ineligible for return. This ineligibility is usually identified during the ordering process, so the pharmacy understands prior to ordering that this drug cannot be returned for credit.

The pharmacy will group together any medications being returned to credit, and the wholesaler provides paperwork for the returns. After receipt of the drugs (and confirming they are not damaged or opened), the wholesaler will apply a credit to the pharmacy account.

Return to Stock (RTS)

In a retail or community pharmacy, prescriptions that have not been picked up in a specified number of days are able to be returned to stock (RTS), or returned to the pharmacy inventory for dispensing to other patients. Pharmacies generally have their own policies regarding the length of time before a return is completed, but usually it is between 7 and 14 days. Pharmacy technicians can help minimize returns by notifying patients they have a prescription ready that needs to be picked up.

Though pharmacies have internal policies regarding the RTS time frame, this may also be dictated by insurance companies providing the drug coverage for the patient. When a prescription is returned to stock, the insurance claim that had processed this prescription is reversed, so the patient's insurance does not pay for a prescription that is not picked up. If this claim is not reversed through the insurance, the pharmacy could still receive the insurance payment, though the patient did not receive the prescription. This would be considered insurance fraud. Insurance companies often define the number of days for return for efficient prescription processing.

When a prescription is returned to stock, it is important that it be kept in the patient's original container. It should never be poured back into the original stock bottle, as it could have a different lot number or expiration date. This bottle is stored on the shelf, with the patient information removed for HIPAA (Health Insurance Portability and Accountability Act of 1996) purposes. The quantity can then be dispensed to another patient, keeping the original expiration date of the prescription returned.

Returns can also occur in an institutional or hospital pharmacy. If a unit dose medication is dispensed to a specific patient, and then that patient is discharged or therapy is discontinued or changed, this unit dose can be returned back to the pharmacy to be used for other patients. The medication must not have been removed from the packaging or have been damaged during the dispensing process.

Reverse Distribution

Outdated or expired medications that cannot be returned to the wholesaler can be sent to a **reverse distributor** for manufacturer credit. A reverse distributor is a vendor who processes expired or damaged medications and removes them from the pharmacy. This often allows pharmacies to receive partial credit back for expired medications. Additionally, the reverse distributor manages the disposal of medications not eligible for credit, which is helpful to the pharmacy. The reverse distributor charges a fee for this process, which is generally deducted from the credit back to the pharmacy.

Medications that are compounded or reconstituted are not eligible for product return. Some manufacturers also may not accept partially used bottles of liquid medication. The reverse distributor can generally accept these and dispose of them properly for the pharmacy in an environmentally safe manner. A reverse distributor will visit the pharmacy to process expired medications, or the pharmacy may be able to ship expired drugs to the reverse distributor. Controlled substances can also be returned using a reverse distributor, as mentioned in Chapter 4.

SUMMING IT UP

- **Compounding** is the process of combining two or more substances to create a product that is not available as a manufactured drug.

- The compounding process cannot occur without the proper equipment and procedures in place. Pharmacy technicians should be familiar with all the terminology and equipment necessary for the compounding process.

- The pharmacy **master formula record (MFR)** is a requirement for USP Chapter <795> and helps to standardize practice. The MFR must contain detailed information about and a specific procedure to follow for each compound. In addition to the MFR, a compounding record must be completed each time compounding takes place.

- Non-sterile medications that are compounded in the pharmacy include the following:

  - **Ointment**—a semisolid mixture that creates a barrier on the skin that provides protection and allows moisture to stay trapped within. A **gel** may also be used for this same purpose.

  - **Emulsion**—a mixture of water and oil, which generally do not mix, but are held together with the use of a stabilizing agent. Creams and lotions are examples of emulsions.

  - A cream can be a **water-in-oil (w/o) emulsion**, which contains more oil than water, or an **oil-in-water (o/w) emulsion**, which contains more water than oil.

  - **Elixir**—a sweet, clear solution containing alcohol.

  - **Solution**—a mixture of liquid and powder in which the powder is completely dissolved.

  - **Suspension**—a mixture of powder and liquid in which the powder is not fully dissolved.

  - **Syrup**—a liquid dosage form sweetened with sugar.

  - **Enema**—a liquid inserted into the rectum through the anus, for the purpose of bowel evacuation.

  - **Suppository**—a solid dosage form that is absorbed through the mucous membranes of the body.

  - **Capsule**—an oral dosage form that is often useful for patients who have difficulty swallowing tablets.

- A calculated **beyond-use date (BUD)** cannot extend past an expiration date of any one of the compounded ingredients.

- Compounding and filling prescriptions require a variety of skills and knowledge of pharmacy calculations and formulas, including fractions, decimals, percentages, ratios and proportions, and dimensional analysis.

- To mix together the same drug in different strengths, an **alligation** can be used to determine how many parts are needed from each ingredient. The final product will have a strength between the two products. Alligations can also be used or to mix a drug with a diluent or inert ingredient to reduce the drug's concentration.

- It is vital to know how to convert among systems of measurement when compounding medications. The systems of measurement from which conversions may be made are as follows:

  - Metric system

  - Household system

  - Apothecary system

  - Celsius to Farenheit

- Pharmacy abbreviations used in prescribing are known as **sig codes**.

- Medical abbreviations for diseases are also used frequently in pharmacy practice.

- The Roman numeral system is used on drug prescriptions to designate quantity or strength and on packaging to designate DEA-assigned schedules for controlled substances.

- Medical terminology is used to understand the meaning of medical words. It consists of one or more root words, prefixes, and suffixes

- **Days' supply** is a calculation that determines how much medicine a patient needs per day. Calculations can be based on either the **total tablets needed** to fill the order or **how many days a quantity will last**.

- Dosage calculations can be solved using ratio proportions and dimensional analysis. In addition, some dosing may be based on weight or on **body surface area (BSA)**.

- Considerations for equipment and supplies related to dispensing medications include the following:

  - Packaging size

  - Unit dose

  - Repacking medications

  - Unit-of-use

  - Durable medical equipment

  - Oral and injectable syringes and needles

- A **lot number** is a number assigned by a manufacturer to a specific batch of drugs produced. Lot numbers are used for tracking purposes by both the manufacturer and the purchaser.

- The **expiration date** of the drug is the last date the manufacturer can guarantee stability, purity, and quality of the medication produced.

- A **National Drug Code (NDC)** number is required for all drugs produced by FDA-registered manufacturers. An NDC number is a unique number comprised of 10 digits, grouped into 3 segments.

- Managing inventory in the pharmacy involves continuous monitoring of expired drugs and utilizing reverse distributors for expired medication credit and prescriptions that can be returned.

PRACTICE QUESTIONS: ORDER ENTRY AND PROCESSING

> **Directions:** Choose the correct answers to the following questions. The answer key and explanations follow the question set.

1. Which of the following has a cylindrical shape with a wide base and is used for liquid measurement, mixing, or heating?

   A. Graduated cylinder

   B. Beaker

   C. Conical cylinder

   D. Mortar and pestle

2. Cocoa butter can be used as a base for melting at body temperature when compounding

   A. ointments.

   B. creams.

   C. enemas.

   D. suppositories.

3. A patient weighs 187 pounds. An order is written for this patient for 8 mg/kg/day in three divided doses. How many mg would there be in one dose?

   A. 227 mg

   B. 499 mg

   C. 680 mg

   D. 1,496 mg

4. Calculate the days' supply for the following prescription:

   ii tabs PO every 4–6 hours PRN disp #36

   A. 2 days

   B. 3 days

   C. 4 days

   D. 7 days

5. A patient has an order written for 135 mL of oral liquid. What size bottle should be used to fill this prescription?

   A. 3 fl. oz.

   B. 4 fl. oz.

   C. 6 fl. oz.

   D. 8 fl. oz.

6. A bulk bottle of oral tablets is repackaged in a hospital pharmacy. The bulk bottle expires in 9 months. What BUD should be documented on these tablets?

   A. The expiration date of the bulk bottle

   B. 30 days

   C. 6 months

   D. 1 year

7. Which of the following is a purpose of the lot number on a medication?

   A. Dosing information

   B. Barcode scanning

   C. Documentation of drug stability

   D. Recall removal

8. The middle set of numbers in an NDC number represents the

   A. manufacturer.

   B. drug.

   C. size of the package.

   D. wholesaler.

9. Prescriptions not picked up by patients should be returned to stock within

   A. 3–5 days.

   B. 7–10 days.

   C. 20–22 days.

   D. 30 days.

10. The process of returning expired or unused medications to a third-party vendor who will process them for credit is known as

    A. reverse distribution.

    B. outdates.

    C. wholesaler credit.

    D. return to stock.

ANSWER KEY AND EXPLANATIONS

1. B	3. A	5. C	7. D	9. B
2. D	4. B	6. C	8. B	10. A

1. **The correct answer is B.** A beaker is used for liquid measurement, mixing, or heating and has a flat edge and wide base. A graduated cylinder (choice A) is a straight-sided measuring device for liquids that comes in different sizes for volume measurements and can be glass or plastic. A conical cylinder (choice C) is a cone-shaped measurement tool that is wider at the top than the bottom and can also be glass or plastic. A mortar (choice D) is a bowl, and a pestle is a tool with a rounded end and handle that is used to crush tablets or triturate powders.

2. **The correct answer is D.** A plant oil, such as cocoa butter, is used for a base when the suppository should melt at body temperature. Ointments (choice A) create a barrier on the skin, and the bases selected are dependent on the use of the ointment as a barrier. Creams (choice B) are designed to absorb into the skin, and the base chosen depends on if the cream is a w/o or o/w compound. Enemas (choice C) are liquids that are administered into the rectum and do not melt, as they are already in liquid form.

3. **The correct answer is A.** Because the patient's weight is given in pounds, and the order is written in mg/kg, the first step is to convert pounds to kg:

$$\frac{187 \text{ lbs.}}{2.2} = 85 \text{ kg}$$

   Next, multiply the patient's kg weight by the mg in the prescribed order:

$$(85 \text{ kg})(8 \text{ mg}) = 680 \text{ mg}$$

   Because the order is written as mg/kg/day, this total represents the patient's daily dose. To determine how many mg in one dose, take the daily dose and divide by 3:

$$\frac{680 \text{ mg}}{3} = 226.66666 = 227 \text{ mg}$$

4. **The correct answer is B.** The order reads "take two tablets by mouth every 4 to 6 hours as needed." To calculate days' supply, assume the patient will take the maximum amount needed. Every 4 hours is equivalent to 6 times daily. If the patient is taking 2 tabs for each dose, (2 tabs)(6 times daily) = 12 tabs is needed for 1 day The order is written for 36 tabs:

$$\frac{x \text{ days}}{36 \text{ tabs}} = \frac{1 \text{ day}}{12 \text{ tabs}}$$

   Cross multiply and divide: $\frac{(36)(1)}{12} = 3$ days.

5. **The correct answer is C.** The bottle size selected should be as close to the volume of the liquid as possible. Six fluid ounces (choice C) would be the appropriate size bottle for this order. A 3 fl. oz. bottle (choice A) would only hold 90 mL, and a 4 fl. oz. bottle (choice B) would only hold 120 mL. An 8 fl. oz. bottle (choice D) would hold 240 mL.

6. **The correct answer is C.** For non-liquid formulations, the BUD for repackaged drugs is 6 months or the expiration date on the bottle, if it is sooner. Since the bulk bottle expiration date is 9 months, a BUD of 6 months should be used.

7. **The correct answer is D.** The lot number is a number assigned by a manufacturer to a specific batch of drugs produced. This lot number is necessary when determining which product is impacted by a recall. It does not provide dosing information (choice A), nor is it utilized for barcode scanning (choice B). The expiration date is used for drug stability information (choice C), not lot numbering.

8. **The correct answer is B.** The middle set of numbers is the product code, which specifies the drug. The first set of numbers is the labeler, most often the manufacturer (choice A). The package size (choice C) is the third set of numbers. Wholesaler information (choice D) is not included in an NDC number.

9. **The correct answer is B.** Prescriptions that have not been picked up by patients should be returned to stock within 7–10 days. This number of days is often dictated by insurance companies to prevent fraud or overpayment of claims. Three to five days (choice A) is often not enough time to pick up prescriptions. Both 20–22 days (choice C) and 30 days (choice D) are too long.

10. **The correct answer is A.** Outdated or expired medications that cannot be returned to the wholesaler can be sent to a reverse distributor for manufacturer credit, known as reverse distribution. Outdates (choice B) is the process of pulling expired medications off the dispensing shelf. Wholesaler credit (choice C) is given after an item is returned. Return to stock (choice D) is returning medications that have not been dispensed to the pharmacy stock.

PART IV
TWO PRACTICE TESTS

ANSWER SHEET PRACTICE TEST 1

1. Ⓐ Ⓑ Ⓒ Ⓓ	19. Ⓐ Ⓑ Ⓒ Ⓓ	37. Ⓐ Ⓑ Ⓒ Ⓓ	55. Ⓐ Ⓑ Ⓒ Ⓓ	73. Ⓐ Ⓑ Ⓒ Ⓓ
2. Ⓐ Ⓑ Ⓒ Ⓓ	20. Ⓐ Ⓑ Ⓒ Ⓓ	38. Ⓐ Ⓑ Ⓒ Ⓓ	56. Ⓐ Ⓑ Ⓒ Ⓓ	74. Ⓐ Ⓑ Ⓒ Ⓓ
3. Ⓐ Ⓑ Ⓒ Ⓓ	21. Ⓐ Ⓑ Ⓒ Ⓓ	39. Ⓐ Ⓑ Ⓒ Ⓓ	57. Ⓐ Ⓑ Ⓒ Ⓓ	75. Ⓐ Ⓑ Ⓒ Ⓓ
4. Ⓐ Ⓑ Ⓒ Ⓓ	22. Ⓐ Ⓑ Ⓒ Ⓓ	40. Ⓐ Ⓑ Ⓒ Ⓓ	58. Ⓐ Ⓑ Ⓒ Ⓓ	76. Ⓐ Ⓑ Ⓒ Ⓓ
5. Ⓐ Ⓑ Ⓒ Ⓓ	23. Ⓐ Ⓑ Ⓒ Ⓓ	41. Ⓐ Ⓑ Ⓒ Ⓓ	59. Ⓐ Ⓑ Ⓒ Ⓓ	77. Ⓐ Ⓑ Ⓒ Ⓓ
6. Ⓐ Ⓑ Ⓒ Ⓓ	24. Ⓐ Ⓑ Ⓒ Ⓓ	42. Ⓐ Ⓑ Ⓒ Ⓓ	60. Ⓐ Ⓑ Ⓒ Ⓓ	78. Ⓐ Ⓑ Ⓒ Ⓓ
7. Ⓐ Ⓑ Ⓒ Ⓓ	25. Ⓐ Ⓑ Ⓒ Ⓓ	43. Ⓐ Ⓑ Ⓒ Ⓓ	61. Ⓐ Ⓑ Ⓒ Ⓓ	79. Ⓐ Ⓑ Ⓒ Ⓓ
8. Ⓐ Ⓑ Ⓒ Ⓓ	26. Ⓐ Ⓑ Ⓒ Ⓓ	44. Ⓐ Ⓑ Ⓒ Ⓓ	62. Ⓐ Ⓑ Ⓒ Ⓓ	80. Ⓐ Ⓑ Ⓒ Ⓓ
9. Ⓐ Ⓑ Ⓒ Ⓓ	27. Ⓐ Ⓑ Ⓒ Ⓓ	45. Ⓐ Ⓑ Ⓒ Ⓓ	63. Ⓐ Ⓑ Ⓒ Ⓓ	81. Ⓐ Ⓑ Ⓒ Ⓓ
10. Ⓐ Ⓑ Ⓒ Ⓓ	28. Ⓐ Ⓑ Ⓒ Ⓓ	46. Ⓐ Ⓑ Ⓒ Ⓓ	64. Ⓐ Ⓑ Ⓒ Ⓓ	82. Ⓐ Ⓑ Ⓒ Ⓓ
11. Ⓐ Ⓑ Ⓒ Ⓓ	29. Ⓐ Ⓑ Ⓒ Ⓓ	47. Ⓐ Ⓑ Ⓒ Ⓓ	65. Ⓐ Ⓑ Ⓒ Ⓓ	83. Ⓐ Ⓑ Ⓒ Ⓓ
12. Ⓐ Ⓑ Ⓒ Ⓓ	30. Ⓐ Ⓑ Ⓒ Ⓓ	48. Ⓐ Ⓑ Ⓒ Ⓓ	66. Ⓐ Ⓑ Ⓒ Ⓓ	84. Ⓐ Ⓑ Ⓒ Ⓓ
13. Ⓐ Ⓑ Ⓒ Ⓓ	31. Ⓐ Ⓑ Ⓒ Ⓓ	49. Ⓐ Ⓑ Ⓒ Ⓓ	67. Ⓐ Ⓑ Ⓒ Ⓓ	85. Ⓐ Ⓑ Ⓒ Ⓓ
14. Ⓐ Ⓑ Ⓒ Ⓓ	32. Ⓐ Ⓑ Ⓒ Ⓓ	50. Ⓐ Ⓑ Ⓒ Ⓓ	68. Ⓐ Ⓑ Ⓒ Ⓓ	86. Ⓐ Ⓑ Ⓒ Ⓓ
15. Ⓐ Ⓑ Ⓒ Ⓓ	33. Ⓐ Ⓑ Ⓒ Ⓓ	51. Ⓐ Ⓑ Ⓒ Ⓓ	69. Ⓐ Ⓑ Ⓒ Ⓓ	87. Ⓐ Ⓑ Ⓒ Ⓓ
16. Ⓐ Ⓑ Ⓒ Ⓓ	34. Ⓐ Ⓑ Ⓒ Ⓓ	52. Ⓐ Ⓑ Ⓒ Ⓓ	70. Ⓐ Ⓑ Ⓒ Ⓓ	88. Ⓐ Ⓑ Ⓒ Ⓓ
17. Ⓐ Ⓑ Ⓒ Ⓓ	35. Ⓐ Ⓑ Ⓒ Ⓓ	53. Ⓐ Ⓑ Ⓒ Ⓓ	71. Ⓐ Ⓑ Ⓒ Ⓓ	89. Ⓐ Ⓑ Ⓒ Ⓓ
18. Ⓐ Ⓑ Ⓒ Ⓓ	36. Ⓐ Ⓑ Ⓒ Ⓓ	54. Ⓐ Ⓑ Ⓒ Ⓓ	72. Ⓐ Ⓑ Ⓒ Ⓓ	90. Ⓐ Ⓑ Ⓒ Ⓓ

Answer Sheet

Practice Test 1

90 Questions—110 minutes

> **Directions:** For each of the following items, choose the correct answer and then fill in the corresponding circle on the answer sheet. Check your answers using the answer key and explanations that follow the test.

1. Which of the following antihypertensive agents is an ARB?

   A. Accupril

   B. Metoprolol

   C. Hydrochlorothiazide

   D. Valsartan

2. A compounded nonaqueous oral solid stored at room temperature has a BUD of

   A. 14 days.

   B. 30 days.

   C. 6 months.

   D. 1 year.

3. Which of the following drugs is considered by the ISMP to be high-risk/high-alert?

   A. Lidocaine patch

   B. Lidocaine cream

   C. Lidocaine continuous infusion

   D. Lidocaine subcutaneous

4. A drug that may or may not have a higher rate of error, but the outcome of an error involving that drug would pose a greater risk to the patient is known as a(n)

   A. LASA medication.

   B. high-alert/high-risk medication.

   C. tall man lettering medication.

   D. error-prone abbreviation.

5. Which of the following is added while compounding to help smoothen the mixture and help any solids to dissolve better?

   A. Levigating agent

   B. Distilled water

   C. Syrup

   D. Cocoa butter

6. Which medication is a neuromuscular blocker?

   A. Enalapril

   B. Propranolol

   C. Sitagliptin

   D. Vecuronium

7. Which of the following drugs is considered by the ISMP to be high-risk/high-alert?

   A. Paroxetine

   B. Doxycycline

   C. Rivaroxaban

   D. Famotidine

8. A patient who takes Cozaar is admitted to the hospital. Which of the following would be an appropriate therapeutic substitution?

   A. Carvedilol

   B. Irbesartan

   C. Enalapril

   D. Clonidine

9. A patient has an order written for 12 fl. oz. of a medication. How many mLs is this?

    A. 120 mL

    B. 180 mL

    C. 240 mL

    D. 360 mL

10. The agency established by OSHA that compiles a list of hazardous drugs is the

    A. EPA.

    B. FDA.

    C. NIOSH.

    D. DEA.

11. Unexpired medications can sometimes be returned to the wholesaler for

    A. reverse distribution.

    B. credit.

    C. RTS.

    D. profit.

12. Which of the following should be disposed of in the sharps container?

    A. Blood products

    B. Empty syringes used when administering chemotherapy

    C. Vials with chemotherapy medication left over from compounding

    D. Ampules used from compounding

13. A patient has a prescription filled, leaves the pharmacy, and after getting home, realizes she gave the pharmacy the wrong prescription. The patient can do which of the following?

    A. Return the medication back to the pharmacy.

    B. Return the medication to the insurance company.

    C. Return the medication to a reverse distributor.

    D. Fill the correct prescription and dispose of the incorrect medication at a drop-off box.

14. In which of the following drug classes is citalopram?

    A. Antidepressant—SNRI

    B. Antidepressant—MAOI

    C. Antidepressant—SSRI

    D. Antidepressant—TCA

15. Which of the following is a muscle relaxant?

    A. Cyclobenzaprine

    B. Methylphenidate

    C. Hydrocodone

    D. Glimepiride

16. A patient fills a 90-day prescription once in 6 months. What is the adherence percentage for this patient?

    A. 25%

    B. 50%

    C. 75%

    D. 100%

17. Which of the following drugs is considered by the ISMP to be high-risk/high-alert?

    A. Risperidone

    B. Solifenacin

    C. Methotrexate

    D. Beclomethasone

18. Which of the following should be used both for compounding hazardous drugs, as well as administering to a patient?

    A. Chemo vial and tubing

    B. PVC-free IV bags

    C. Closed-system transfer device (CTSD)

    D. CADD pump

19. Some medications are written containing uppercase, bolded letters to draw attention to the differences in drug names; this practice is known as

    A. confused drug alert.

    B. high-risk medications.

    C. tall man lettering.

    D. five rights.

20. An order is written for a chemotherapy medication for 2 mg/kg. The patient's weight is 168 pounds. What is the dose for this patient?

    A. 124.9 mg

    B. 138.7 mg

    C. 143.8 mg

    D. 152.7 mg

21. Oral contraceptives packaged in a 28-day supply are which type of medication?

    A. Unit dose

    B. Repackaged

    C. Unit-of-use

    D. Nebulizer

22. A patient receives a prescription for amoxicillin suspension on March 1st. What would the BUD be for this suspension?

    A. March 8

    B. March 11

    C. March 15

    D. March 29

23. A patient is prescribed a dose of 20 mg/kg. The patient weighs 110 pounds. How many grams will be in each dose?

    A. 2.2 g

    B. 1000 g

    C. 2200 g

    D. 1 g

24. Which of the following chapters defines safe handling of hazardous drugs?

    A. USP Chapter <795>

    B. USP Chapter <797>

    C. USP Chapter <800>

    D. USP Chapter <1160>

25. What does the second letter in a prescriber's DEA number represent?

    A. The prescriber's level of practice

    B. The first letter of the prescriber's first name

    C. The first letter of the prescriber's last name

    D. The first letter of the month of birth of the prescriber

26. Dicyclomine is which type of drug?

    A. Antispasmodic

    B. Antidepressant

    C. Muscle relaxant

    D. Corticosteroid

27. Magnesium sulfate can be mistaken for which drug?

    A. Triamcinolone

    B. Morphine sulfate

    C. Methotrexate

    D. Compazine

28. USP Chapter <797> requires that the walls, ceiling, and shelves of the clean room be cleaned at what frequency?

    A. Daily

    B. Twice daily (open and close)

    C. Monthly

    D. Every 6 months

29. A patient has a prescription for lorazepam 0.5 mg PO TID PRN #30. What is the days' supply for this order?

    A. 5 days

    B. 7 days

    C. 10 days

    D. 15 days

30. Tramadol is available as a

    A. 10 mg capsule.

    B. 25 mg liquid.

    C. 50 mg tablet.

    D. 250 mg suspension.

31. Which drug must be swallowed with 8 ounces of plain water immediately after rising for the day and must be taken 30 minutes before first food, beverage, or medication of the day?
    A. Levothyroxine
    B. Metformin
    C. Ethinyl estradiol and desogestrel
    D. Alendronate

32. A vial of Pneumovax is good for how many days after withdrawing the first dose?
    A. 6 hours
    B. 28 days
    C. 42 days
    D. Manufacturer expiration date

33. Which type of syringe ranges in volume from 3 mL to 60 mL and can be used to administer oral doses?
    A. Insulin
    B. Tuberculin
    C. Hypodermic
    D. Filter

34. An abbreviation for which of the following drugs may be mistaken as hydrocortisone?
    A. Propylthiouracil
    B. TNKase
    C. Hydrochlorothiazide
    D. Magnesium sulfate

35. Which of the following is a fast-acting insulin?
    A. Insulin glargine
    B. Insulin human
    C. Insulin aspart
    D. Insulin detemir

36. Levothyroxine is available in which strength and dosage forms?
    A. 1 mg–10 mg tablets
    B. 100 mg–200 mg injection
    C. 5 g oral suspension
    D. 25 mcg–300 mcg tablets

37. How often must a Schedule II inventory be conducted?
    A. Monthly
    B. Initially, and annually thereafter
    C. Initially, and biennially thereafter
    D. Initially, and every 3 years thereafter

38. A pharmacy technician adds 10 mL of a stock solution into 200 mL of water. What is the percent v/v?
    A. 3%
    B. 5%
    C. 10%
    D. 20%

39. A patient with tachycardia has
    A. a slow heart rate.
    B. low blood pressure.
    C. high blood pressure.
    D. a fast heart rate.

40. Which schedule of controlled substance includes medications that may be purchased without a prescription?
    A. Schedule II
    B. Schedule III
    C. Schedule IV
    D. Schedule V

41. A 9% w/v solution has how many grams of active ingredient?
    A. 9 mg
    B. 9 g
    C. 0.9 g
    D. 90 mg

42. Which medication is most likely to be misused?
    A. Allopurinol
    B. Loratadine
    C. Methylphenidate
    D. Spironolactone

43. Zanaflex is the name brand of
    A. temazepam.
    B. tizanidine.
    C. timolol.
    D. triamcinolone.

44. Venlafaxine is in which drug class?
    A. Antidepressant—SSRI
    B. Antidepressant—SNRI
    C. Antidepressant—TCA
    D. Antidepressant—MAOI

45. When a patient is prescribed numerous medications, this is known as
    A. geriatric pharmacy.
    B. polypharmacy.
    C. Beers List.
    D. ADE.

46. A pharmacy technician is calculating how many days' supply is written for a prescription. The order is written as Take 1 cap PO QID PRN disp 28. The technician calculates this as a 10-day supply because the order is written for PRN. Which type of error would this be?
    A. Prescribing error—prescriptions cannot be written QID PRN
    B. Dispensing error—this would not last the patient 10 days
    C. Administering error—the patient should not be taking medications PO
    D. Monitoring error—the patient should not be taking a medication QID

47. Which schedule of controlled substances is generally used for antitussive, analgesic, and antidiarrheal purposes?
    A. Schedule II
    B. Schedule III
    C. Schedule IV
    D. Schedule V

48. A patient is getting a heparin bolus dosed at 3500 units. Heparin is available as a 5000 units/mL vial. How many mL are in the bolus dose?
    A. 0.7 mL
    B. 1.2 mL
    C. 1.4 mL
    D. 2.8 mL

49. Oxybutynin is used for
    A. hormone replacement.
    B. hyperlipidemia.
    C. overactive bladder.
    D. bacterial infection.

50. Which of the following must be true in order for a drug to be considered a therapeutic equivalent?
    A. The drug must be issued a B code.
    B. The drug must be in tablet form only.
    C. The drug must use the same dosage and route of administration.
    D. The drug must not be considered bioequivalent.

51. A recall that is unlikely to cause any adverse reaction, but which violates FDA standards for safety and efficacy is which type of recall?
    A. Class I
    B. Class II
    C. Class III
    D. Class IV

52. A HEPA filter must be certified every
    A. 14 days.
    B. 30 days.
    C. 6 months.
    D. 1 year.

Practice Test 1

53. Which of the following is used to reduce intraocular pressure in patients with glaucoma or ocular hypertension?

   A. Fluticasone

   B. Bacitracin; Neomycin; Polymyxin B

   C. Erythromycin

   D. Timolol

54. The generic name for Restoril is

   A. carbamazepine.

   B. zolpidem.

   C. temazepam.

   D. venlafaxine.

55. Lotrel is a combination antihypertensive agent that contains benazepril and which other drug?

   A. Propranolol

   B. Lisinopril

   C. Verapamil

   D. Amlodipine

56. If the pharmacy counter was disinfected, what kind of cleaning has occurred?

   A. Reduction in number of microbes

   B. Decontamination of hazardous drugs

   C. Killing of all microbials

   D. Blood-borne pathogen prevention

57. A prescription is written for 150 mL. Which of the following size bottles should be used to fill this prescription?

   A. 3 fl. oz.

   B. 4 fl. oz.

   C. 6 fl. oz.

   D. 12 fl. oz.

58. How many times can a prescription for controlled substance Schedules III–V be transferred?

   A. None—no transfers permitted

   B. Once

   C. As many times as refills remaining

   D. Only if the pharmacies are within the same chain

59. A technician is counting amoxicillin tablets that have left a white residue on the counting tray. If the technician continues to the next prescription without cleaning the tray, what may occur?

   A. Nothing—there is no cross-sensitivity with amoxicillin

   B. Cross contamination and potential patient harm

   C. Development of a penicillin allergy

   D. Development of a cephalosporin allergy

60. A drug-drug interaction in which the effects of the drugs are essentially "summed" together is which type of effect?

   A. Additive

   B. Potentiation

   C. Synergistic

   D. Antagonistic

61. Mometasone is which type of drug?

   A. Corticosteroid

   B. Bronchodilator

   C. Leukotriene inhibitor

   D. Antitussive

62. Intuniv is the name brand of

   A. methylprednisolone.

   B. dextromethorphan.

   C. methotrexate.

   D. guanfacine.

63. A medication error that is caught before it reaches the patient is known as a(n)

   A. adverse drug event.

   B. adverse drug reaction.

   C. contraindication.

   D. near miss.

64. Which of the following requirements for the DSCSA includes information dating back to the original manufacturing of the product?

A. Transaction history

B. Transaction information

C. Transaction wholesaler

D. Transaction statement

65. A patient taking St. John's wort who is also prescribed fluoxetine could experience which type of interaction?

A. Drug-disease

B. Drug-laboratory

C. Drug-dietary supplement

D. Drug-nutrient

66. A day designated by the FDA for patients to dispose of unused medications is called

A. reverse distribution.

B. drop off.

C. take-back.

D. needle disposal.

67. If a hood or PEC has been shut off prior to compounding, how long must it be run before using?

A. 10 minutes

B. 15 minutes

C. 30 minutes

D. 60 minutes

68. Which dosage form contains a substance that reacts with water to give off carbon dioxide and, as a result, causes a fizz?

A. Buccal

B. Sublingual

C. Enteric-coated

D. Effervescent

69. Which dosage form is solid at room temperature but designed to melt and release medication in the body?

A. Suppository

B. Enema

C. MDI

D. Irrigation

70. A nebule is given via which route of administration?

A. Transdermal

B. Injection

C. Ophthalmic

D. Inhalation

71. A reaction that causes a painful red or purple rash that spreads and blisters and can be a result of taking ibuprofen, acetaminophen, or penicillin is

A. Reye's syndrome.

B. Stevens-Johnson syndrome.

C. impetigo.

D. photosensitivity.

72. A refrigerator containing vaccines must have temperatures logged how frequently?

A. Once daily

B. Twice daily

C. Once per week

D. Every hour

73. Which of the following is the proper order for garbing in PPE?

A. Hair cover, shoe covers, sterile gloves, gown

B. Shoe covers, face mask, gown, gloves, hair cover

C. Sterile gloves, gown, shoe covers, face mask

D. Shoe covers, hair cover, face mask, gown, sterile gloves

74. Insulin glargine is stable for how many days after opening?

A. 7 days

B. 14 days

C. 28 days

D. 42 days

75. Which of the following may be used during non-sterile compounding?

A. Stirring rod

B. CSTD

C. Regular needle

D. CAI

76. A pharmacy technician is entering a prescription for a patient. The prescription reads, Metformin 50 mg, take 1 tablet QD for BP. The pharmacy technician notices this is an error. What type of error would this be?

A. Indication error

B. Dispensing error

C. Administration error

D. Monitoring error

77. Which of the following is a method of mitigating adverse events in a REMS program?

A. Requiring laboratory testing to monitor effects

B. Providing psychiatric counseling for patients taking any medication in the REMS program

C. Ensuring patients work exclusively with their physician and not a pharmacist or other provider

D. Keeping warning labels minimal to avoid inducing panic to patients

78. Which medication is used for a UTI?

A. Warfarin

B. Nitrofurantoin

C. Celecoxib

D. Conjugated estrogens

79. Cetirizine is indicated to treat

A. cough.

B. congestion.

C. production of mucus.

D. allergic rhinitis.

80. Which of the following would require restricted access, with accessibility limited to pharmacy staff only?

A. Frequently used medications

B. 0.9% sodium chloride

C. Concentrated electrolytes

D. Crash carts

81. Which of the following can help prevent an administration error?

A. CPOE

B. Tall man lettering

C. Vital signs

D. BCMA

82. A patient is getting ready to take a cruise and mentions to the pharmacist that she gets sea sick easily. The pharmacist might mention which herbal supplement as a possible treatment for motion sickness?

A. Echinacea

B. Ginger

C. Chamomile

D. Valerian

83. Which of the following pseudoephedrine purchases would be allowed under the CMEA?

A. Purchasing 8 boxes at 1.5 grams each in a 30-day period

B. Purchasing 12 boxes at 0.5 grams each in one day

C. Purchasing 6 boxes at 2 grams each in a 30-day period

D. Purchasing 3 boxes with 0.4 g in each on one day

84. Vitamin B$_{12}$ is also known as
   A. niacin.
   B. riboflavin.
   C. folic acid.
   D. cyanocobalamin.

85. Which antibiotic has a 5–10% chance of a cross-sensitivity reaction with penicillin?
   A. Levofloxacin
   B. Sulfamethoxazole-trimethoprim
   C. Azithromycin
   D. Cephalexin

86. A patient has a documented allergy to sulfa, and the prescriber calls in an order for Bactrim. Which type of error is this?
   A. Prescribing error
   B. Dispensing error
   C. Administration error
   D. Monitoring error

87. Which of the following may cause edema, flushing, headache, and fatigue?
   A. Venlafaxine
   B. Atorvastatin
   C. Diltiazem
   D. Albuterol

88. Decongestants, such as pseudoephedrine, cause which side effects?
   A. Drowsiness and sedation
   B. Hypotension and shortness of breath
   C. Nervousness, excitability, dizziness, and insomnia
   D. Headache and low blood sugar

89. MedWatch is a reporting system through which organization?
   A. FDA
   B. ISMP
   C. DEA
   D. AHRQ

90. An example of an emulsion would be a(n)
   A. solution.
   B. enema.
   C. cream.
   D. ointment.

Practice Test 1

Answers Practice Test 1

ANSWER KEY AND EXPLANATIONS

1. D	16. B	31. D	46. B	61. A	76. A
2. C	17. C	32. D	47. D	62. D	77. A
3. C	18. C	33. C	48. A	63. D	78. B
4. B	19. C	34. C	49. C	64. A	79. D
5. A	20. D	35. C	50. C	65. C	80. C
6. D	21. C	36. D	51. C	66. C	81. D
7. C	22. C	37. C	52. C	67. C	82. B
8. B	23. D	38. B	53. D	68. D	83. D
9. D	24. C	39. D	54. C	69. A	84. D
10. C	25. C	40. D	55. D	70. D	85. D
11. B	26. A	41. B	56. C	71. B	86. A
12. D	27. B	42. C	57. C	72. B	87. C
13. D	28. C	43. B	58. B	73. D	88. C
14. C	29. C	44. B	59. B	74. C	89. A
15. A	30. C	45. B	60. A	75. A	90. C

1. **The correct answer is D.** Valsartan has the suffix given to all ARBS, -*sartan*. Accupril (choice A) is an ACE inhibitor (-*pril*), metoprolol (choice B) is a beta blocker (-*olol*), and hydrochlorothiazide (choice C) is a thiazide diuretic (-*thiazide*).

2. **The correct answer is C.** USP Chapter <795> has guidelines for calculating BUDs. A nonaqueous oral solid stored at room temperature is stable for 6 months. Aqueous dosage forms (emulsions, gels, creams, solutions, sprays, or suspensions) that are refrigerated are good for 14 days and nonaqueous dosage forms (suppositories, ointments) stored at room temperature are good for 90 days.

3. **The correct answer is C.** Antiarrhythmic IV infusions are considered high-risk, but only in that dosage form. A lidocaine patch, cream, or subcutaneous injection would not be considered high-risk.

4. **The correct answer is B.** High-alert/high-risk medications have a heightened risk of harm if used in error. LASA (choice A) drugs are those that look alike and sound alike. Tall man lettering (choice C) is used to help highlight differences in medications that look similar. Error-prone abbreviations (choice D) are those that, when used, are more likely to cause an error.

5. **The correct answer is A.** A levigating agent may be used to smoothen a preparation or help a solid compound dissolve better. It is generally a viscous liquid, such as mineral oil. Distilled water (choice B) is used for reconstitution but does not help smoothen the mixture. A syrup (choice C) is sugar-based liquid that is not used for levigating. Cocoa butter (choice D) is a base for suppositories, but it does not help levigate.

6. **The correct answer is D.** Neuromuscular blockers end with a suffix of *–curium* or *–curonium*. Enalapril (choice A) is an ACE inhibitor, and propranolol (choice B) is a beta blocker. Sitagliptin (choice C) is used for diabetes treatment.

7. **The correct answer is C.** Antithrombotic agents, including direct oral anticoagulants such as rivaroxaban, are on the ISMP high-risk/high-alert medication list. Paroxetine (choice A), doxycycline (choice B), and famotidine (choice D) are not considered high-risk medications.

8. **The correct answer is B.** Therapeutic substitution occurs when a medication is substituted for another in the same drug class. Cozaar is an ARB and would be interchanged for irbesartan. Carvedilol (choice A) is a beta blocker, enalapril (choice C) is an ACE inhibitor, and clonidine (choice D) is an alpha agonist.

9. **The correct answer is D.** To convert fl. oz. to mL, multiply by 30. (12)(30) = 360 mL. 120 mL (choice A) would be 4 fl. oz., 180 mL (choice B) would be 6 fl. oz., and 240 mL (choice C) would be 8 fl. oz.

10. **The correct answer is C.** The National Institute for Occupational Safety and Health (NIOSH), whose mission is to conduct research and make recommendations in regard to employee and workplace safety, completes a list of hazardous drugs. The EPA (choice A) is responsible for environmental protection issues. The FDA (choice B) approves new drugs and oversees the recall process. The DEA (choice D) is responsible for controlled substance regulation.

11. **The correct answer is B.** Unexpired and approved medication may be returned to the wholesaler for credit. A third party does reverse distribution (choice A)—not a pharmacy wholesaler. RTS (choice C) is a process in which prescriptions that have not been picked up in a specified number of days are able to be returned to stock or returned to the pharmacy inventory for dispensing to other patients. A profit (choice D) cannot occur when medications are returned to the wholesaler—the pharmacy is not selling these back but rather is returning them for credit.

12. **The correct answer is D.** Ampules must be broken upon use, and the broken glass should be disposed of in the sharps container. Blood products (choice A) should be disposed of in a red biohazard container. Empty syringes used for hazardous drug administration such as chemotherapy (choice B) are disposed of in a yellow chemotherapy container. Vials with medication remaining (choice C) should be disposed of in a black hazardous waste container.

13. **The correct answer is D.** If a prescription medication is given to a patient and leaves the pharmacy, it cannot be returned or re-dispensed. Once a drug has been out of the possession of the pharmacy, it cannot be verified for purity, quality, or strength. The patient must dispose of this incorrect medication if necessary and have the correct prescription filled.

14. **The correct answer is C.** Citalopram (Celexa) is an SSRI that blocks the reuptake of serotonin, which increases levels of serotonin in the brain. SNRIs (choice A) block the reuptake of both serotonin and norepinephrine, increasing the levels of both neurotransmitters in the brain. MAOIs (choice B) inhibit monoamine oxidate, which increases levels of neurotransmitters in the brain. TCAs (choice D) inhibit reuptake of serotonin and norepinephrine, which increases levels of both neurotransmitters and inhibits action of acetylcholine.

15. **The correct answer is A.** Cyclobenzaprine (Flexeril) is a muscle relaxant. Methylphenidate (choice B) is a stimulant and a controlled substance. Hydrocodone (choice C) is a narcotic analgesic and a controlled substance. Glimepiride (choice D) is an antidiabetic medication.

16. **The correct answer is B.** Adherence can be calculated as a percentage using the total days' supply for all patient fills divided by the total days in a given period.

$$\text{Adherence Percentage} =$$

$$\frac{\text{Total Days' Supply of Patient Fills}}{\text{Total Days}} \times 100$$

If a patient filled a medication for a 90-day supply just once in 6 months, this would be 90 days of total therapy divided by 180 days of total time.

$$6 \text{ months} \times 30\frac{\text{days}}{\text{month}} = 180 \text{ total days}$$

$$\frac{90 \text{ total days' supply}}{180 \text{ total days}} \times 100 = 50\%$$

17. **The correct answer is C.** Oral methotrexate is a specific drug considered by the ISMP to be high-risk/high-alert. Risperidone (choice A), solifenacin (choice B), and beclomethasone (choice D) are not considered high-risk drugs.

18. **The correct answer is C.** The purpose of a CSTD is to provide a greater level of protection to health care workers who are compounding and administering a hazardous drug to a patient. Chemo vial and tubing (choice A) is used for compounding, but the vial is not used when administering. PVC-free IV bags (choice B) are necessary only when the medication has a physical incompatibility with PVC—not all hazardous drugs require PVC-free bags. A CADD pump (choice D) is used to deliver chemotherapy to patients over an extended period of time.

19. **The correct answer is C.** Tall man lettering helps emphasize the parts of the drug name that are not the same, to distinguish between look-alike/sound-alike medications, and help prevent medication errors. Confused drug alerts (choice A) are not a published alert, although facility EMRs may have these. High-risk medications (choice B) are on a list produced by the ISMP. The "five rights" (choice D) are patient rights for safe medication administration.

20. **The correct answer is D.** First, the pounds must be converted into kilograms:

$$\frac{168 \text{ lbs.}}{2.2} = 76.4 \text{ kg}$$

Next, set up a ratio proportion. This problem can also be solved by multiplying the mg dose by the total kg of the patient:

$$\frac{x\,\text{mg}}{76.4\,\text{kg}} = \frac{2\,\text{mg}}{1\,\text{kg}}$$

Solve for x:

$$x = (76.4)(2) = 152.7 \text{ mg}$$

21. **The correct answer is C.** A unit-of-use package is a medication that is labeled in the original manufacturer container, which contains sufficient quantity for a course of therapy. Unit dose (choice A) is a manufactured single dose of a medication. A repackaged medication (choice B) results from using a bulk bottle to produce individual unit doses. A nebulizer (choice D) is a machine used for respiratory treatments.

22. **The correct answer is C.** Amoxicillin suspension has a stability of 14 days, which means the BUD is 14 days from the date it was reconstituted. March 8 (choice A) would be 7 days, March 11 (choice B) would be 10 days, and March 29 (choice D) would be a 28-day BUD. These are all incorrect dating.

23. **The correct answer is D.** First, start by converting the pounds to kilograms by dividing by 2.2:

$$\frac{110}{2.2} = 50 \text{ kg}$$

Because the dose is 20 mg/kg, this means the patient is taking 20 mg for every kg. To solve for the total for this dose, multiply 20 mg by 50 kg:

$$(20)(50) = 1,000 \text{ mg}$$

Because the question is looking for grams, the answer in mg must be converted. To convert mg to g, divide by 1,000 or move the decimal place 3 places to the left:

$$\frac{1,000 \text{ mg}}{1,000} = 1 \text{ g}$$

24. **The correct answer is C.** USP Chapter <800> defines standards for safe handling of hazardous drugs to minimize exposure to both patients as well as healthcare workers. USP Chapter <795> (choice A) defines standards for non-sterile compounding. USP Chapter <797> (choice B) defines standards for sterile compounding. USP Chapter <1160> (choice D) provides guidance for pharmaceutical calculations in prescription compounding.

25. **The correct answer is C.** A DEA number consists of two letters followed by seven digits. The first letter of the DEA number is either A, B, F, or M, depending on the prescriber's level of practice. The second letter is the first letter of the prescriber's last name (choice C). The remaining numbers are a formula designed by the DEA to deter diversion.

26. **The correct answer is A.** Dicyclomine is an antispasmodic. It is not an antidepressant (choice B), muscle relaxant (choice C), or corticosteroid (choice D).

27. **The correct answer is B.** The abbreviation used for magnesium sulfate is $MgSO_4$, and morphine sulfate is MSO_4. These are often confused and should be written out. Triamcinolone (choice A), methotrexate (choice C), and compazine (choice D) should all be written out, but are not generally confused with magnesium sulfate.

28. **The correct answer is C.** In an institutional pharmacy, USP Chapter <797> requires a monthly cleaning of walls, ceilings, and any shelves located in the buffer and ante room. This cleaning must be documented on a monthly log. Daily and twice daily (choices A and B) are not required frequencies, and every 6 months (choice D) is not often enough.

29. **The correct answer is C.** The directions read as 1 tablet by mouth three times daily as needed. The patient could take a maximum of 3 tablets daily, and the total quantity dispensed is 30 tablets.

$$\frac{30 \text{ tabs}}{3 \text{ tabs per day}} = 10 \text{ days}$$

30. **The correct answer is C.** Tramadol is available in 50 mg, 100 mg, and 200 mg tablets. There is no capsule, oral liquid, or suspension form of tramadol.

31. **The correct answer is D.** Alendronate is a bisphosphonate which must be swallowed with 8 ounces of plain water immediately after rising for the day and must be taken 30 minutes before first food, beverage, or medication of the day. Patients should be able to stand or sit upright for 30 minutes after taking. Levothyroxine (choice A), metformin (choice B), and ethinyl estradiol and desogestrel (choice C) should all be taken in the morning but do not have the same requirements as alendronate.

32. **The correct answer is D.** After a vial of Pneumovax is opened, it can be used until the manufacturer's listed expiration date.

33. **The correct answer is C.** Hypodermic syringes are typically plastic syringes that range in size from 3 mL to 60 mL. These syringes can also be used for oral administration. Insulin syringes (choice A) are used for insulin administration to diabetic patients. These syringes are size 1 mL or less and are measured in both mL and units for insulin dosing. Tuberculin syringes (choice B) are small syringes that hold up to 1 mL and are used for intradermal administration of a purified protein derivative (PPD). There are no filter syringes (choice D), but filter needles are used for drawing up medication from an ampule.

34. **The correct answer is C.** Hydrochlorothiazide is often abbreviated as HCTZ and can be misread as hydrocortisone. It is not mistaken for propylthiouracil (choice A), TNKase (choice B), or magnesium sulfate (choice D).

35. **The correct answer is C.** Insulin aspart is a fast-acting insulin. Insulin glargine (choice A) and insulin detemir (choice D) are both long-acting insulins. Insulin human (choice B) is an intermediate insulin.

36. **The correct answer is D.** Levothyroxine is dosed in mcg tablet form and available in dosage strengths of 25 mcg–300 mcg. It is not available in 1mg–10mg tablets (choice A), a 100 mg–200mg injection (choice B), or a 5 g oral suspension (choice C).

37. **The correct answer is C.** A Schedule II inventory must be completed at initial registration and every two years thereafter. The Schedule II inventory must be an accurate, physical count, while the Schedule III–V inventory may be estimated. Inventory records must be kept for a minimum of two years, and the Schedule II inventory must be separated from the Schedule III–V inventory.

38. **The correct answer is B.** Start by using the ratio proportion method to calculate. In this problem, we do not know the percent concentration, but can find it based on the new stock formula and using 100 mL as our base percentage.

$$\frac{x\,\text{mL}}{100\,\text{mL}} = \frac{10\,\text{mL}}{200\,\text{mL}}$$

Dimensional analysis can also be used:

$$\frac{10\,\text{mL}}{200\,\text{mL}} \,\bigg|\, 100\,\text{mL}$$

Both methods are solved by

$$\frac{(10)(100)}{200} = 5\,\text{mL} = \frac{5\,\text{mL}}{100\,\text{mL}} = 5\%.$$

39. **The correct answer is D.** *Tachy-* is the prefix meaning "fast," and *cardio-* is the root word for *heart*. A slow heart rate (choice A) would be bradycardia, low BP (choice B) is hypotension, and high BP (choice C) is hypertension.

40. **The correct answer is D.** There are some Schedule V medications that may also be purchased without a prescription. Pharmacies are often required to log this information and limit to patients who are 18 years of age or older. Schedule II, III, and IV medications must have a prescription for dispensing.

41. **The correct answer is B.** Percent weight/volume (w/v) describes the number of grams in 100 mL of a solution. A 9% solution would be 9 grams in 100 mL.

42. **The correct answer is C.** Misuse may be due to non-compliance or drug abuse. CNS stimulants, such as methylphenidate, are more frequently misused. Allopurinol (choice A), loratadine (choice B), and spironolactone (choice D) are not medications often misused.

43. **The correct answer is B.** Zanaflex is the name brand of tizanidine. Temazepam (choice A) is the generic of Restoril, timolol (choice C) is the generic of Timoptic, and triamcinolone (choice D) is the generic for Kenalog.

44. **The correct answer is B.** Venlafaxine is an SNRI, which blocks the reuptake of serotonin and norepinephrine, increasing levels of serotonin in the brain. SSRIs (choice A) block the reuptake of serotonin, increasing the level of serotonin in the brain. TCAs (choice C) inhibit reuptake of serotonin and norepinephrine, which increases levels of both neurotransmitters and inhibits action of acetylcholine. MAOIs (choice D) inhibit monoamine oxidate, which increases levels of neurotransmitters in the brain.

45. **The correct answer is B.** If a patient is taking numerous medications, this is known as polypharmacy. Geriatrics (choice A) may pose a higher risk of ADE and are more susceptible to disease-drug interactions and often require adjusted dosing for renal failure. The Beers List (choice C) is used to identify medications and classes of medications which may be inappropriate for geriatric use. An ADE (choice D) is an injury caused by a drug.

46. **The correct answer is B.** A dispensing error can result from calculation errors, incorrect patient selection, or inappropriate refills, such as refills too soon (early refill). A patient taking a medication QID PRN is 4 times daily. If 28 capsules are dispensed with 4 being taken each day, this is a 7-day supply only. There is no information to tell if the order is written incorrectly, and the patient has not yet administered or monitored this medication.

47. **The correct answer is D.** Schedule V controlled substances have little abuse potential (less than Schedule IV) and are generally used for antitussive, analgesic, and antidiarrheal purposes. Schedule II–IV are not always used for these purposes.

48. **The correct answer is A.** To solve, use a ratio-proportion. Set up a ratio proportion:

$$\frac{x\,\text{mL}}{3,500\,\text{units}} = \frac{1\,\text{mL}}{5,000\,\text{units}}$$

Solve for x.

$$x\,\text{mL} = \frac{(3,500)(1)}{5,000}$$
$$x = 0.7\,\text{mL}$$

49. **The correct answer is C.** Oxybutynin is used to treat overactive bladder. It is not used for hormone replacement (choice A), hyperlipidemia (choice B), or a bacterial infection (choice D).

50. **The correct answer is C.** For a drug to be considered therapeutically equivalent, the following criteria must be met:

- Approved for safety and effectiveness
- Contains the same active ingredients (pharmaceutical equivalence)
- Uses the same route of administration
- Elicits same effect with same dosage
- Meets the same standards for purity, quality, and strength
- Processed in the body in the same way as the original drug (bioequivalent)
- Manufactured with good manufacturing practices (GMP)

Drugs issued a B code are not therapeutically equivalent. The dosage form does not need to be a tablet, and the drug must be considered bioequivalent.

51. **The correct answer is C.** A Class III recall is one issued for a medicine that is unlikely to cause any adverse action but which violates FDA standards for safety and efficacy. A Class I recall (choice A) is a recall for a medication that if used could cause serious health problems or death. A Class II recall (choice B) is a recall for a medication that might cause a temporary health problem if used, or causes a slightly serious threat and no immediate danger but risk of injury is present. There is no Class IV (choice D) recall.

52. **The correct answer is C.** The HEPA filter for all PECs must be certified every six months. Fourteen and thirty days are not necessary, and one year would be out of compliance.

53. **The correct answer is D.** Timolol is an ophthalmic solution used to reduce intraocular pressure in patients with glaucoma or ocular hypertension. Fluticasone is used for asthma and COPD; bacitracin, neomycin, polymyxin B, and erythromycin all are used for ophthalmic infection caused by bacteria.

Answers Practice Test 1

Answers Practice Test 1

54. **The correct answer is C.** The name brand of temazepam is Restoril. Tegretol is the name brand for carbamazepine (choice A), Ambien is the name brand of zolpidem (choice B), and Effexor is the name brand of venlafaxine (choice D).

55. **The correct answer is D.** Lotrel contains both benazepril and amlodipine. It does not contain propranolol (choice A), lisinopril (choice B), or verapamil (choice C).

56. **The correct answer is C.** Disinfecting kills microbials. Sanitizing reduces the number of microbes present (choice A). Disinfecting does not decontaminate hazardous drugs (choice B) or prevent blood-borne pathogens (choice D).

57. **The correct answer is C.** 1 fl. oz. is equal to 30 mL, so 6 fl. oz. is equal to 180 mL. When selecting package size, it's important to get as close to the volume as possible, without overfill. 3 fl. oz. (choice A) would be 90 mL, and 4 fl. oz. (choice B) would be 120 mL, which would not be big enough for 150 mL. 12 fl. oz. (choice D) would be 360 mL, which would be too big for this volume.

58. **The correct answer is B.** A Schedule III, IV, or V prescription may be transferred to another pharmacy once only. Unlimited transfers are not permitted. This rule does exempt pharmacies that share electronic databases, such as those within pharmacy chains, but a transfer does not have to be within the same chain.

59. **The correct answer is B.** Cross contamination occurs when a medication has left a residue that contaminates the next medication being counted. This can be dangerous for patients who have a serious allergy to a medication; if any residue remains following the counting of one of these drugs, and contaminates the next patient's prescription, the patient could suffer an allergic reaction. There is cross-sensitivity with penicillin antibiotics and cephalosporins, although this

is not relevant for the question. A patient cannot develop an allergy from residue exposure.

60. **The correct answer is A.** Summation or an additive interaction occurs when the effect of two drugs is the same as the effect each drug would have if taken individually; essentially the "sum" of taking the drugs together. Potentiation (choice B) is an interaction that causes one drug to prolong or increase the effect of another drug. Synergism (choice C) is an interaction in which the combined effect of two drugs is much larger or longer in duration than the sum of the two. Antagonism (choice D) occurs when the interaction between two drugs causes one drug to work against the other.

61. **The correct answer is A.** Mometasone is a corticosteroid that can be used intranasally. It does not dilate the bronchioles or inhibit leukotrienes and is not an antitussive agent.

62. **The correct answer is D.** The generic of Intuniv is guanfacine. Methylprednisolone (choice A) is the generic of Medrol, dextromethorphan (choice B) is the generic of Delsym, and methotrexate (choice C) is the generic of Trexall.

63. **The correct answer is D.** A medication error that is caught before it reaches the patient is known as a near miss. Near misses are as important to monitor, identify, and report as medication errors. These events help identify trends in potential errors, workflow concerns, and prescribing issues. If a drug error harms a patient, this is considered an adverse drug event (choice A). An adverse drug reaction (choice B) is a reaction to a medication that may be either preventable or non-preventable. A contraindication (choice C) is a situation or disease state that makes a therapy unadvisable.

64. **The correct answer is A.** Transaction history (TH) includes transaction information going back to the original manufacturing of the product. Transaction information (choice B) is the name, strength, dosage form, NDC, container size, number of containers purchased, lot number, date of purchase and shipment, and business name of address purchasing. There is no transaction wholesaler (choice C) included in the DSCSA. The transaction statement (choice D) is a statement that declares that the the manufacturer did not knowingly ship a counterfeit or illegitimate product, has systems in place for proper procedure, and did not knowingly alter any transaction history.

65. **The correct answer is C.** St. John's wort used for OTC depression treatment can modify neurotransmitters in the brain, which can disrupt the action of SSRIs. A drug-disease interaction (choice A) can occur if a patient's disease alters the absorption, metabolism, or elimination of a drug. A drug-laboratory interaction (choice B) is caused by medications that may impact laboratory results and cause false positives or negatives when testing. A drug-nutrient interaction (choice D) may include those found in food or beverages which may interact with medications.

66. **The correct answer is C.** Patients may dispose of controlled substances (and other expired or unused medications) through take-back programs, which are designated days sponsored by the DEA. A take-back day allows patients to dispose of any unwanted medications in a safe manner and helps patients clean out medication cabinets to prevent inadvertent drug abuse or misuse.

67. **The correct answer is C.** If the PEC has been shut off at any time, it should be run for 30 minutes before use.

68. **The correct answer is D.** An effervescent tablet is one that contains a substance (such as sodium bicarbonate) which reacts with water to give off carbon dioxide (and causes a fizz) and must be dissolved before administration. A buccal tablet (choice A) is placed between the gums and the cheek and dissolves. A sublingual tablet (choice B) is placed under the tongue and dissolves. Enteric-coated tablets (choice C) are designed to prevent dissolving in the stomach, and intended to bypass and dissolve in the intestine.

69. **The correct answer is A.** A suppository is a dosage form which melts at body temperature when inserted and delivers medication into the body. An enema (choice B) is a liquid injected into the rectum for bowel cleansing or to deliver medication. A metered dose inhaler, or MDI (choice C), is used to deliver a fixed quantity of drug into the lungs when inhaled properly. An irrigation (choice D) is used to wash wounds, the bladder, or the eyes.

70. **The correct answer is D.** A nebule is a small vial of fluid used with a nebulizer to deliver medication into the lungs via inhalation. The transdermal route of administration (choice A) generally involves a patch delivering medication through the skin. An injection (choice B) is a route of administration which bypasses the intestines. And the ophthalmic route of administration (choice C) is via the eye.

71. **The correct answer is B.** Stevens-Johnson syndrome consists of painful red or purple rash that spreads and blisters, and is caused by allopurinol, acetaminophen, ibuprofen, penicillin, or anticonvulsants. Reye's syndrome (choice A) is a serious condition involving swelling in the brain and liver damage that can occur in children receiving aspirin. Impetigo (choice C) is a highly contagious skin infection. Photosensitivity (choice D) is a side effect of many drugs which causes patients to burn more easily in the sun.

72. **The correct answer is B.** If a refrigerator contains vaccines, the temperature must be logged twice daily. Once daily and per week are not frequent enough for measuring vaccines and once every hour is excessive for required measurement.

73. **The correct answer is D.** Shoe covers are donned first and next a hair cover and beard cover, if needed, should be donned, along with a face mask. Next a non-shedding gown is donned over clean scrubs, followed by sterile gloves. Hand washing and hand hygiene are completed during this process.

74. **The correct answer is C.** Insulin glargine (Lantus) is stable for 28 days after opening and must be discarded after this time. It is still stable after 7 and 14 days, but does not last for 42 days.

75. **The correct answer is A.** A glass stirring rod may be used when stirring substances that need to be dissolved or mixed thoroughly. CSTD, needles, and a CAI are all used during sterile compounding and have different requirements for PPE and sterility.

76. **The correct answer is A.** Prescribing errors may also include indication errors. Lack of drug knowledge may cause an error in prescribing due to contraindication or abnormal doses. Metformin is available as a 500 mg tablet, not 50 mg, and is used to treat diabetes, not blood pressure. The medication was not dispensed or administered, so this not a dispensing, administration, or monitoring error.

77. **The correct answer is A.** REMS can help mitigate adverse events through clinical interventions, such as education on specific risks, communication programs, and requiring laboratory testing to monitor effects. Psychiatric counseling, though beneficial to some patients on REMS medications, is not provided through the REMS program. Pharmacists play an integral part in the REMS program and should not be excluded from this process. Warning labels are published in medication guides to help educate patients and prevent possible side effects.

78. **The correct answer is B.** Nitrofurantoin (Macrobid) is used for treatment of a UTI. Warfarin (choice A) is an anticoagulant. Celecoxib (choice C) is used for rheumatoid arthritis, osteoarthritis, management of acute pain, and dysmenorrhea. Conjugated estrogens (choice D) are used for hormone replacement.

79. **The correct answer is D.** Cetirizine is an antihistamine used for treatment of allergic rhinitis. It is not used for cough (choice A), congestion (choice B), or production of mucus (choice C).

80. **The correct answer is C.** Medications with restricted accessibility include concentrated electrolytes because they must be diluted prior to administration. Medications that are frequently used (choice A) will be stocked in a dispensing cabinet or floor stock for nursing access and ease of use; 0.9% sodium chloride (choice B) may be stocked in central supply or nursing units for fluid administration. Crash carts (choice D) must not be restricted to pharmacy staff only, as these may be needed in the event of an emergency.

81. **The correct answer is D.** Administration errors can be prevented through the use of BCMA. Patient's wristbands are scanned to prevent administration to the wrong patient. Scanning the drug prior to dispensing also helps identify if the drug is incorrect, including the route, dose, and dosage form. CPOE (choice A) would help mitigate prescribing errors, tall man lettering (choice B) would help prevent dispensing errors, and noting vital signs (choice C) would help mitigate monitoring errors.

82. **The correct answer is B.** Ginger can be used for nausea and motion sickness treatment. Echinacea (choice A) is used for immune system support, and chamomile (choice C) is a sedative or calming agent. Valerian (choice D) is used for insomnia or anxiety treatment.

83. **The correct answer is D.** CMEA set specific requirements and restrictions for pseudoephedrine purchases, which are limited to 3.6 grams daily or 9 grams in a 30-day period. Purchasing 3 boxes at 0.4 g each equals 1.2 gram total in one day, which is under the allowed limit. Purchasing 8 boxes at 1.5 grams each (choice A) equals 12

grams in 30 days, which is over the allowed limit. Purchasing 12 boxes at 0.5 grams each (choice B) equals 6 grams in one day, which is over the allowed limit. Purchasing 6 boxes at 2 grams each (choice C) equals 12 grams in 30 days, which is over the allowed limit.

84. **The correct answer is D.** Vitamin B_{12} is also known as cyanocobalamin. Vitamin B_3 is niacin (choice A), vitamin B_2 is riboflavin (choice B), and vitamin B_9 is folic acid (choice C).

85. **The correct answer is D.** The cephalosporin class of antibiotics has a 5–10% chance of hypersensitivity in patients with penicillin allergies. Levofloxacin (choice A) is a fluoroquinolone, sulfamethoxazole-trimethoprim (choice B) is a sulfa drug, and azithromycin (choice C) is a macrolide antibiotic, so these will not result in cross sensitivity.

86. **The correct answer is A.** A prescribing error occurs when there is an error in the written order from the prescriber. This could occur through the prescribing of a medication that is inappropriate based on patient allergies or other contraindications. If this patient is allergic to sulfa, Bactrim would be contraindicated for therapy. Dispensing errors (choice B) occur after the prescription has been filled or patient has received the order. Administration errors (choice C) occur upon administration, and a monitoring error (choice D) would occur after administration.

87. **The correct answer is C.** Calcium channel blockers such as Diltiazem can cause edema, flushing, headache, and fatigue as side effects. Venlafaxine (choice A) can cause nausea, dry mouth, constipation, insomnia, decreased appetite, or diarrhea. Atorvastatin (choice B) can cause constipation, muscle pain, or dyspepsia. Albuterol (choice D) can cause nausea, vomiting, nervousness, headache, insomnia, or palpitations.

88. **The correct answer is C.** Decongestants stimulate the CNS, causing excitability and insomnia. They do not cause drowsiness and may increase blood pressure (not hypotension). They do not typically cause a headache, and do not reduce blood sugar.

89. **The correct answer is A.** The FDA has a reporting system for adverse and safety events known as MedWatch. ISMP (choice B) has a medication error reporting system known as MERP. The DEA (choice C) regulates controlled substances but does not have a medication error reporting system. AHRQ (choice D) is the Agency for Healthcare Research and Quality and reviews medication errors for potential trends in practice.

90. **The correct answer is C.** An emulsion is a mixture of water and oil, which generally does not mix, but which is held together with the use of a stabilizing agent. Creams and lotions are examples of emulsions. A solution (choice A) is a mixture of liquid and powder in which the powder is completely dissolved. An enema (choice B) is a type of solution, administered into the rectum through the anus. An ointment (choice D) is a semisolid mixture that contains the highest oil content of the topical dosage forms.

ANSWER SHEET PRACTICE TEST 2

1. Ⓐ Ⓑ Ⓒ Ⓓ   19. Ⓐ Ⓑ Ⓒ Ⓓ   37. Ⓐ Ⓑ Ⓒ Ⓓ   55. Ⓐ Ⓑ Ⓒ Ⓓ   73. Ⓐ Ⓑ Ⓒ Ⓓ
2. Ⓐ Ⓑ Ⓒ Ⓓ   20. Ⓐ Ⓑ Ⓒ Ⓓ   38. Ⓐ Ⓑ Ⓒ Ⓓ   56. Ⓐ Ⓑ Ⓒ Ⓓ   74. Ⓐ Ⓑ Ⓒ Ⓓ
3. Ⓐ Ⓑ Ⓒ Ⓓ   21. Ⓐ Ⓑ Ⓒ Ⓓ   39. Ⓐ Ⓑ Ⓒ Ⓓ   57. Ⓐ Ⓑ Ⓒ Ⓓ   75. Ⓐ Ⓑ Ⓒ Ⓓ
4. Ⓐ Ⓑ Ⓒ Ⓓ   22. Ⓐ Ⓑ Ⓒ Ⓓ   40. Ⓐ Ⓑ Ⓒ Ⓓ   58. Ⓐ Ⓑ Ⓒ Ⓓ   76. Ⓐ Ⓑ Ⓒ Ⓓ
5. Ⓐ Ⓑ Ⓒ Ⓓ   23. Ⓐ Ⓑ Ⓒ Ⓓ   41. Ⓐ Ⓑ Ⓒ Ⓓ   59. Ⓐ Ⓑ Ⓒ Ⓓ   77. Ⓐ Ⓑ Ⓒ Ⓓ
6. Ⓐ Ⓑ Ⓒ Ⓓ   24. Ⓐ Ⓑ Ⓒ Ⓓ   42. Ⓐ Ⓑ Ⓒ Ⓓ   60. Ⓐ Ⓑ Ⓒ Ⓓ   78. Ⓐ Ⓑ Ⓒ Ⓓ
7. Ⓐ Ⓑ Ⓒ Ⓓ   25. Ⓐ Ⓑ Ⓒ Ⓓ   43. Ⓐ Ⓑ Ⓒ Ⓓ   61. Ⓐ Ⓑ Ⓒ Ⓓ   79. Ⓐ Ⓑ Ⓒ Ⓓ
8. Ⓐ Ⓑ Ⓒ Ⓓ   26. Ⓐ Ⓑ Ⓒ Ⓓ   44. Ⓐ Ⓑ Ⓒ Ⓓ   62. Ⓐ Ⓑ Ⓒ Ⓓ   80. Ⓐ Ⓑ Ⓒ Ⓓ
9. Ⓐ Ⓑ Ⓒ Ⓓ   27. Ⓐ Ⓑ Ⓒ Ⓓ   45. Ⓐ Ⓑ Ⓒ Ⓓ   63. Ⓐ Ⓑ Ⓒ Ⓓ   81. Ⓐ Ⓑ Ⓒ Ⓓ
10. Ⓐ Ⓑ Ⓒ Ⓓ   28. Ⓐ Ⓑ Ⓒ Ⓓ   46. Ⓐ Ⓑ Ⓒ Ⓓ   64. Ⓐ Ⓑ Ⓒ Ⓓ   82. Ⓐ Ⓑ Ⓒ Ⓓ
11. Ⓐ Ⓑ Ⓒ Ⓓ   29. Ⓐ Ⓑ Ⓒ Ⓓ   47. Ⓐ Ⓑ Ⓒ Ⓓ   65. Ⓐ Ⓑ Ⓒ Ⓓ   83. Ⓐ Ⓑ Ⓒ Ⓓ
12. Ⓐ Ⓑ Ⓒ Ⓓ   30. Ⓐ Ⓑ Ⓒ Ⓓ   48. Ⓐ Ⓑ Ⓒ Ⓓ   66. Ⓐ Ⓑ Ⓒ Ⓓ   84. Ⓐ Ⓑ Ⓒ Ⓓ
13. Ⓐ Ⓑ Ⓒ Ⓓ   31. Ⓐ Ⓑ Ⓒ Ⓓ   49. Ⓐ Ⓑ Ⓒ Ⓓ   67. Ⓐ Ⓑ Ⓒ Ⓓ   85. Ⓐ Ⓑ Ⓒ Ⓓ
14. Ⓐ Ⓑ Ⓒ Ⓓ   32. Ⓐ Ⓑ Ⓒ Ⓓ   50. Ⓐ Ⓑ Ⓒ Ⓓ   68. Ⓐ Ⓑ Ⓒ Ⓓ   86. Ⓐ Ⓑ Ⓒ Ⓓ
15. Ⓐ Ⓑ Ⓒ Ⓓ   33. Ⓐ Ⓑ Ⓒ Ⓓ   51. Ⓐ Ⓑ Ⓒ Ⓓ   69. Ⓐ Ⓑ Ⓒ Ⓓ   87. Ⓐ Ⓑ Ⓒ Ⓓ
16. Ⓐ Ⓑ Ⓒ Ⓓ   34. Ⓐ Ⓑ Ⓒ Ⓓ   52. Ⓐ Ⓑ Ⓒ Ⓓ   70. Ⓐ Ⓑ Ⓒ Ⓓ   88. Ⓐ Ⓑ Ⓒ Ⓓ
17. Ⓐ Ⓑ Ⓒ Ⓓ   35. Ⓐ Ⓑ Ⓒ Ⓓ   53. Ⓐ Ⓑ Ⓒ Ⓓ   71. Ⓐ Ⓑ Ⓒ Ⓓ   89. Ⓐ Ⓑ Ⓒ Ⓓ
18. Ⓐ Ⓑ Ⓒ Ⓓ   36. Ⓐ Ⓑ Ⓒ Ⓓ   54. Ⓐ Ⓑ Ⓒ Ⓓ   72. Ⓐ Ⓑ Ⓒ Ⓓ   90. Ⓐ Ⓑ Ⓒ Ⓓ

Answer Sheet

Practice Test 2

90 Questions—110 minutes

Directions: For each of the following items, choose the correct answer and then fill in the corresponding circle on the answer sheet. Check your answers using the answer key and explanations that follow the test.

---

1. Which medication is a local anesthetic?

   A. Lidocaine

   B. Fluconazole

   C. Montelukast

   D. Donepezil

2. When a prescription is returned to stock in a pharmacy, what happens to the insurance claim?

   A. It is maintained for pharmacy profit.

   B. The claim is reversed.

   C. The pharmacy must notify the insurance company for a prior authorization.

   D. The patient must pay cash the next time the prescription is filled.

3. Which of the following capsule sizes is the smallest, holding approximately 50 mg?

   A. 5

   B. 2

   C. 1

   D. 00

4. If the drug class for citalopram was indicated as an abbreviation on a prescription, what might it be confused with?

   A. Acetaminophen

   B. Morphine sulfate

   C. Hydrochlorothiazide

   D. Sliding scale regular insulin

5. Which of the following organizations publishes a high-alert/high-risk medication list for internal pharmacy use?

   A. FDA

   B. DEA

   C. NIOSH

   D. ISMP

6. Many medications in the antiviral drug class end in

   A. *–cillin.*

   B. *–vir.*

   C. *–sporin.*

   D. *–toin.*

7. Which of the following organizations defines what makes a drug hazardous and maintains a hazardous drug list?

   A. FDA

   B. NIOSH

   C. SDS

   D. DEA

8. An order is written for 100 mL of a 6% solution. You have a 10% solution in stock. How much stock solution and how much diluent are needed to compound this order?

   A. 50 mL stock, 50 mL diluent

   B. 20 mL stock, 80 mL diluent

   C. 60 mL stock, 40 mL diluent

   D. 70 mL stock, 30 mL diluent

9. Which of the following should always be disposed of in a red biohazard container?

   A. Infectious waste

   B. Needles

   C. Gowns and gloves used when compounding chemotherapy

   D. Warfarin packaging

10. Which of the following drugs is considered by the ISMP to be high-risk/high-alert?

    A. Glimepiride

    B. Clindamycin

    C. Meclizine

    D. Ipratropium

11. A patient's insurance is requiring an alternative generic medication to the prescribed fexofenadine. Which of the following would be an appropriate therapeutic substitution?

    A. Pseudoephedrine

    B. Benzonatate

    C. Loratadine

    D. Guaifenesin

12. How much dextrose is in a 250 mL bag of D5W?

    A. 10 g

    B. 12.5 g

    C. 15 g

    D. 20 g

13. Which of the following is used to measure the weight of an item or substance using a Class A balance?

    A. Weighing paper

    B. Vehicle

    C. Beaker

    D. Calibration weights

14. Which of the following vaccines should be stored frozen?

    A. Hepatitis A

    B. Rotavirus

    C. Varicella

    D. Pneumococcal

15. Which of the following is able to be used for several doses?

    A. SDV

    B. Ampule

    C. MDV

    D. Epidural

16. Which of the following drugs is considered by the ISMP to be high-risk/high-alert?

    A. Apixaban

    B. Bupropion

    C. Citalopram

    D. Aripiprazole

17. What is the maximum number of refills that could be written for a prescription for hydromorphone?

    A. No refills

    B. 1 refill

    C. 5 refills in 6 months

    D. No restriction on refills

18. A patient has a 30-day supply of medication that is filled 8 times in one year. What is the adherence percentage for this patient?

    A. 25%

    B. 33%

    C. 56%

    D. 66%

19. The abbreviation for International Unit is often confused with

    A. U.

    B. IM.

    C. TPN.

    D. IV.

20. Which of the following is the appropriate way to write "nine milligrams"?

    A. 9.0 mg

    B. 9 mcg

    C. 9 mg

    D. 9.0 mcg

21. A pharmacy technician needs to prepare 100 grams of 3% hydrocortisone ointment using 5% and 1% hydrocortisone base. How many grams of each are required to compound this order?

    A. 60 g of the 1% and 40 g of the 5%

    B. 70 g of the 1% and 30 g of the 5%

    C. 50 g of the 1% and 50 g of the 5%

    D. 75 g of the 1% and 25 g of the 5%

22. A patient has an order written as "Take 1 tablet PO QAM DX HTN." The patient is taking a medication for

    A. heartburn.

    B. headache.

    C. high cholesterol.

    D. blood pressure.

23. The first set of numbers of an NDC represent the

    A. labeler.

    B. drug.

    C. package size.

    D. lot number.

24. A patient uses the first dose from his regular insulin vial on April 1st. What BUD should he apply to this vial?

    A. April 15

    B. April 29

    C. May 13

    D. The expiration date on the vial

25. A patient has an order for a medication for 200 mg/m². The patient has a BSA of 1.1 m². What is the total dose for this patient in mg?

    A. 220 mg

    B. 225 mg

    C. 230 mg

    D. 2,250 mg

26. Which of the following are PPE that may be worn in the pharmacy to prevent hazardous drug exposure?

    A. Lab coat

    B. Isolation kit

    C. Shoe covers and gloves

    D. Radiation dosimetry badge

27. Which of the following DEA forms is needed when destroying outdated or damaged controlled substances?

    A. DEA Form 41

    B. DEA Form 106

    C. DEA Form 222

    D. DEA Form 224

28. Benzonatate is which type of drug?

    A. Decongestant

    B. Antihistamine

    C. Antitussive

    D. Expectorant

29. Celebrex is available in 100 mg and 200 mg

    A. tablets.

    B. capsules.

    C. oral solutions.

    D. IV injections.

30. A patient is prescribed Levemir 13 units subQ TID. A 10 mL vial of insulin contains 100 units/mL. How long will one vial of insulin last?

    A. 14 days

    B. 25 days

    C. 38 days

    D. 76 days

31. Which of the following is used for at-home testing of blood glucose?

    A. Coagulation analyzer

    B. Glucometer

    C. Salivary assay

    D. Pulse oximeter

32. The process of reviewing clinical interventions for potential changes to patient therapy for optimal outcomes is known as

    A. adherence.

    B. medication reconciliation.

    C. drug utilization review.

    D. therapeutic substitution.

33. Which of the following drugs stimulates insulin release from beta cells in the pancreas and increases sensitivity of tissues to insulin?

    A. Metformin

    B. Furosemide

    C. Prednisone

    D. Levothyroxine

34. Which of the following statements is true regarding receiving controlled substances in the pharmacy?

    A. Each line of a Schedule II invoice can be signed by a pharmacy technician.

    B. Schedule III and IV medications must be locked in a vault with Schedule II narcotics.

    C. The pharmacist must sign each line of a Schedule II invoice.

    D. The pharmacy technician can document how many Schedule II packages are received on the invoice.

35. Which of the following ISO levels would consist of the dirtiest air?

    A. ISO 5

    B. ISO 6

    C. ISO 7

    D. ISO 8

36. A patient has an order for a medication for 15 mg/m². The patient has a BSA of 1.6 m². The medication is available as a 100 mg/5 mL vial. How many mL is needed per dose?

    A. 1.2 mL

    B. 3.4 mL

    C. 3.8 mL

    D. 4.2 mL

37. Schedule II narcotics must be stored

    A. in an open matrix drawer in an ADC.

    B. on the regular shelves in a pharmacy inventory.

    C. in an unlocked floor stock on a nursing unit.

    D. within a vault or safe in the pharmacy.

38. Which syringe would be measured in mL and units?

    A. Insulin

    B. Tuberculin

    C. Hypodermic

    D. Ampule

39. What is the drug class of lamotrigine?

    A. Antifungal agent

    B. Antihistamine

    C. Antidiabetic

    D. Anticonvulsant

40. Therapeutic equivalence is identified in the FDA Orange Book as which code?

    A. A

    B. B

    C. C

    D. D

41. Which of the following is included as an ADE?

    A. Adverse drug reactions

    B. Near miss

    C. Polypharmacy

    D. Therapeutic substitution

42. Which of the following is required on a prescription for a controlled substance?

    A. Patient's known allergies

    B. Prescriber DEA number

    C. Pharmacy phone number

    D. Patient's medical record number

43. A prospective DUR is performed

    A. before the medication is dispensed.

    B. after the patient has received the medication.

    C. when the patient refills the prescription.

    D. when the patient is being prescribed the medication.

44. Janumet is a combination diabetic agent that contains metformin and which drug?

    A. Glipizide

    B. Sitagliptin

    C. Liraglutide

    D. Glyburide

45. Which medication is considered to have a narrow therapeutic index?

    A. Clindamycin

    B. Triamcinolone

    C. Levothyroxine

    D. Rosuvastatin

46. A patient has a prescription for 3 tsp TID PO × 7d. Select the correct package size that would be most appropriate to fill this order.

    A. 125 mL

    B. 250 mL

    C. 360 mL

    D. 480 mL

47. A patient has a prescription for levothyroxine 75 mcg. How many mg is this dose?

    A. 7.5 mg

    B. 750 mg

    C. 0.75 mg

    D. 0.075 mg

48. When cleaning a CAI, what must also be cleaned in addition to the main compounding chamber?

    A. Buffer chamber

    B. HEPA filter

    C. Glove box

    D. Antechamber

49. Humira is indicated for treatment of

    A. nodular acne.

    B. psoriasis and Crohn's disease.

    C. impetigo.

    D. athlete's foot, jock itch, and ringworm.

50. Robaxin is the name brand of

    A. carisoprodol.

    B. methocarbamol.

    C. chlorthalidone.

    D. brimonidine.

51. A pharmacy technician is entering an order for tramadol 50 mg for a patient. The order is written as 1 tab PO Q4–6HPRN DISP#24. The technician calculates this as a 6-day supply. What type of error is this?

    A. Prescribing error—tramadol should not be taken every 4 to 6 hours

    B. Dispensing error—this would last the patient 4 days

    C. Administering error—the patient may be misusing this medication

    D. Monitoring error—the patient should avoid tramadol for allergies

52. Hydralazine is used to treat

    A. high cholesterol.

    B. high blood pressure.

    C. diabetes.

    D. inflammation.

Practice Test 2

53. An order is written for 1,000 mL of a 4% solution. You have a 12% solution in stock. How much stock solution and how much diluent are needed to compound this order?

   A. 333 mL diluent is added to 667 mL stock

   B. 700 mL diluent is added to 300 mL stock

   C. 400 mL diluent is added to 600 mL stock

   D. 667 mL diluent is added to 333 mL stock

54. Which of the following is used to compound hazardous drugs?

   A. CAI

   B. CACI

   C. Horizontal flow hood

   D. HEPA

55. A drug with the suffix –oxacin is in which drug class?

   A. Steroid

   B. Antibiotic

   C. Antiviral

   D. Antihyperlipidemic

56. Which of the following questions should be considered when conducting an RCA?

   A. What is an appropriate level of punishment for the error that occurred?

   B. What are all the possible human errors that caused this event?

   C. What can we do to prevent it from happening again?

   D. How badly was the patient harmed from the error?

57. How many times can a prescription for a Schedule II controlled substance be transferred?

   A. None—no transfers permitted

   B. Once

   C. As many times as refills remaining

   D. Unlimited if the pharmacies are within the same chain

58. A drug-drug interaction in which the effects of the drug are greater or longer in duration than the sum of the two is which type of effect?

   A. Additive

   B. Potentiation

   C. Synergistic

   D. Antagonistic

59. CPOE helps prevent medication errors by

   A. utilizing confusing abbreviations.

   B. transcribing verbal orders.

   C. preventing the dispensing of an expired medication.

   D. eliminating manual writing of prescriptions.

60. Which of the following needles is the smallest?

   A. 15 G

   B. 19 G

   C. 25 G

   D. 30 G

61. Which ISO level is required for clean air flow within a PEC?

   A. ISO class 5

   B. ISO class 6

   C. ISO class 7

   D. ISO class 8

62. Lansoprazole is indicated to treat

   A. GERD.

   B. high cholesterol.

   C. rhinitis.

   D. nausea and vomiting.

63. A patient taking rosuvastatin should avoid drinking which beverage for potential interaction?
    A. Milk
    B. Tea
    C. Coffee
    D. Grapefruit juice

64. Which dosage form is designed to dissolve under the tongue?
    A. Buccal
    B. Sublingual
    C. Enteric-coated
    D. Effervescent

65. How often should hood cleaning occur?
    A. At the end of the day only
    B. At the beginning of every shift and after a batch is completed
    C. Every 60 minutes
    D. At the beginning of every shift, every 30 minutes or before every batch, and if a spill occurs

66. If a medication is injected into the top layer of the skin, this would be considered which route of administration?
    A. Intra-arterial
    B. Intradermal
    C. Intravenous
    D. Intramuscular

67. Which route of administration involves the delivery of medication systemically through the skin?
    A. Otic
    B. Transdermal
    C. Parenteral
    D. IV push

68. Which of the following may be used to measure the exact volume of a liquid?
    A. Mortar
    B. Weigh boat
    C. Graduated cylinder
    D. Ointment slab

69. Which of the following may result if aspirin is administered to a child?
    A. Reye's syndrome
    B. Stevens-Johnson syndrome
    C. Tendon rupture
    D. Tooth decay and discoloration

70. Which of the following best describes an automated dispensing cabinet?
    A. A cabinet that dispenses IVs only for nurses to administer to patients
    B. A cabinet located in a patient's room for medication withdrawal
    C. A cabinet located securely in a nursing unit for dispensing of frequently used medications
    D. A cabinet used in the pharmacy for dispensing of medications by technicians.

71. At which stage in the garbing process should hand washing occur?
    A. After the sterile gloves have been donned
    B. After the non-shedding gown has been donned
    C. After shoe covers and a hair cover are donned
    D. Before donning any type of PPE

72. Which of the following must be used quickly after opening, as the contents are exposed to air?
    A. SDV
    B. MDV
    C. Insulin vial
    D. Ampule

73. Which of the following medications would require a med guide?

  A. Atorvastatin

  B. Atenolol

  C. Meloxicam

  D. Lisinopril

74. A patient with a cold and a secondary viral infection is prescribed cefdinir. Which of the following best describes this prescription error?

  A. Underuse

  B. Overuse

  C. Misuse

  D. Administration error

75. Benzonatate is indicated for relief of

  A. rhinitis.

  B. congestion.

  C. fever.

  D. cough.

76. Which of the following may have a side effect of pain at the injection site?

  A. Adalimumab

  B. Loperamide

  C. Methylcellulose

  D. Clonazepam

77. A prescriber does not view a critical lab result for a patient and, as a result, the patient suffers drug toxicity from impaired renal function. This would be an example of which type of error?

  A. Prescribing error

  B. Dispensing error

  C. Administration error

  D. Monitoring error

78. What is the purpose of a desiccant?

  A. To protect a medication from light degradation

  B. To protect a medication from heat exposure

  C. To protect a medication from physical incompatibilities

  D. To protect a medication from moisture accumulation

79. For which of the following is ginseng indicated?

  A. Energy boost

  B. BPH

  C. Insomnia

  D. Migraine

80. Which vitamin is important for blood clotting?

  A. Vitamin A

  B. Vitamin D_2

  C. Vitamin E

  D. Vitamin K

81. A patient taking which medication should avoid sunlight?

  A. Bactrim

  B. Tegretol

  C. Percocet

  D. Lantus

82. Spironolactone would cause a significant interaction with which drug?

  A. Metoprolol

  B. Verapamil

  C. Losartan

  D. Enalapril

83. Which of the following could be used to prevent a dispensing error?

  A. CPOE

  B. Barcode scanning

  C. Monitoring creatinine levels

  D. Using the "five rights"

84. Which of the following storage ranges would be appropriate for carbidopa/levodopa?
    A. 2°C to 8°C
    B. 8°C to 15°C
    C. 20°C to 25°C
    D. 30°C to 40°C

85. Meloxicam is available in which strengths and dosage forms?
    A. 100 mg and 200 mg capsules
    B. 50 mg tablets
    C. 7.5 mg and 15 mg tablets
    D. 75 mg cream

86. Which class of drugs should be taken in the morning?
    A. HMG-CoA reductase inhibitors
    B. Beta blockers
    C. Diuretics
    D. Hypnotics

87. Unexpected bleeding could be a side effect of which of the following?
    A. Vitamin K
    B. Bactrim DS
    C. Claritin
    D. Coumadin

88. Which of the following error reporting tools may initiate a recall by the FDA?
    A. MERP
    B. AHRQ
    C. MedWatch
    D. RCA

89. The process of creating smaller particles through crushing, grinding, or pulverizing using a mortar and pestle is known as
    A. trituration.
    B. levigation.
    C. spatulation.
    D. geometric dilution.

90. An order is written for 250 mL of a 2% solution. You have a 6% solution in stock. How much stock solution and how much diluent are needed to compound this order?
    A. 166.7 mL diluent is added to 83.3 mL stock.
    B. 200 mL diluent is added to 50 mL stock.
    C. 142.8 mL diluent is added to 107.2 mL stock.
    D. 151.7 mL diluent is added to 98.3 mL stock.

ANSWER KEY AND EXPLANATIONS

Answers Practice Test 2

1. A	16. A	31. B	46. C	61. A	76. A
2. B	17. A	32. C	47. D	62. A	77. D
3. A	18. D	33. A	48. D	63. D	78. D
4. D	19. D	34. C	49. B	64. B	79. A
5. D	20. C	35. D	50. B	65. D	80. D
6. B	21. C	36. A	51. B	66. B	81. A
7. B	22. D	37. D	52. B	67. B	82. D
8. C	23. A	38. A	53. D	68. C	83. B
9. A	24. B	39. D	54. B	69. A	84. C
10. A	25. A	40. A	55. B	70. C	85. C
11. C	26. C	41. A	56. C	71. C	86. C
12. B	27. A	42. B	57. A	72. D	87. D
13. D	28. C	43. A	58. C	73. C	88. C
14. C	29. B	44. B	59. D	74. B	89. A
15. C	30. B	45. C	60. D	75. D	90. A

1. **The correct answer is A.** Lidocaine is a local anesthetic and can be identified by the suffix –*caine* in the drug name. Fluconazole (choice B) is an antifungal agent, montelukast (choice C) is an antiasthmatic/antiallergy agent, and donepezil (choice D) is used for treatment of Alzheimer's.

2. **The correct answer is B.** When a prescription is returned to stock, the insurance claim that processed this prescription is reversed so that the patient's insurance does not pay for a prescription that is not picked up. It cannot be maintained for profit (choice A), as that would be fraud. The pharmacy does not need to call for a prior authorization (choice C), and the patient does not need to pay cash the next time the prescription is filled (choice D).

3. **The correct answer is A.** The sizes of capsules range from 5 (smallest) to 000 (largest), so 5 would be the smallest, able to hold on average 50 mg of medication.

4. **The correct answer is D.** Citalopram is an SSRI, and if this abbreviation is used, it may be confused with sliding scale regular insulin. The abbreviation used for acetaminophen (choice A) is APAP, morphine sulfate (choice B) is MSO_4, and hydrochlorothiazide (choice C) is HCTZ.

5. **The correct answer is D.** The main purpose of the Institute for Safe Medication Practices (ISMP) is to develop tools and research to prevent medication errors. One way to help prevent errors is identifying specific medications and categories of medications which have a heightened risk of harm if used in error. The FDA (choice A) has an approved drug list with requirements for tall man lettering and is responsible for overall drug approval and safety. The DEA (choice B) regulates controlled substances, and NIOSH (choice C) is the organization that identifies hazardous drugs.

6. **The correct answer is B.** Antiviral medications, such as oseltamivir, end with the suffix *–vir*. Penicillin antibiotics end in *–cillin*, and *–sporin* is used for immunosupressants, such as cyclosporine. Some antiepileptic drugs end in *–toin*.

7. **The correct answer is B.** The National Institute for Occupational Safety and Health (NIOSH) defines what makes a drug hazardous and maintains a hazardous drug list. The FDA (choice A) approves new drugs and oversees the recall process. An SDS (choice C) is a safety data sheet, which provides information on safe handling of hazardous drugs. The DEA (choice D) is responsible for controlled substance regulation.

8. **The correct answer is C.**

   $C_1 = 10$
   $V_1 = x$
   $C_2 = 6$
   $V_2 = 100$

   $$(C_1)(V_1) = (C_2)(V_2)$$

   $$(10)(x) = (6)(100)$$

   Solve for x.

   $$\frac{600}{10} = 60$$

   60 mL of stock is needed.

   To calculate the volume of diluents needed, subtract the stock volume from total volume:

   $$100 \text{ mL} - 60 \text{ mL} = 40 \text{ mL diluent}$$

9. **The correct answer is A.** Red biohazard containers are used for biohazard waste disposal, which includes blood, bodily fluid, and infectious wastes. Needles (choice B) must be disposed of in the sharps container. Gowns and gloves used for chemotherapy compounding (choice C) should go in the yellow chemotherapy container. Warfarin packaging (choice D) should be disposed of in the hazardous waste container.

10. **The correct answer is A.** Sulfonylurea hypoglycemic agents, including glimepiride, are on the ISMP high-risk/high-alert medication list. Clindamycin, meclizine, and ipratropium are not considered high-risk medications.

11. **The correct answer is C.** Therapeutic substitution occurs when a medication is substituted for another in the same drug class. Fexofenadine is an antihistamine, which could be therapeutically interchanged for loratadine. Pseudoephedrine (choice A) is a decongestant, benzonatate (choice B) is an antitussive, and guaifenesin (choice D) is an expectorant.

12. **The correct answer is B.** Dextrose w/v = 5%, or 5 grams dextrose in 100 mL water.

    To determine the total amount of dextrose in 500 mL, set up a ratio proportion:

    $$\frac{x \text{ grams}}{250 \text{ mL}} = \frac{5 \text{ grams}}{100 \text{ mL}}$$

    Solve for x:

    $$\frac{(250)(5)}{100}$$

    $$x = 12.5 \text{ g}$$

13. **The correct answer is D.** Calibration weights are used to measure the weight of a substance in a class A balance. Weighing paper (choice A) is disposable paper that holds a small amount of powder or substance when weighing. A vehicle (choice B) is an inactive or inert substance into which the active ingredient can be mixed into, and a beaker (choice C) is used for liquid measurement, mixing, or heating.

14. **The correct answer is C.** All live vaccines must be stored frozen. Varicella (chicken pox) must be stored in the freezer. Hepatitis A, rotavirus, and pneumococcal vaccines can all be stored in the refrigerator.

Answers Practice Test 2

15. **The correct answer is C.** A multi-dose vial (MDV) can be used for several different doses if it is not punctured within a patient treatment area. Single-dose vials (SDV) and ampules do not contain preservatives and must not be used more than once. An epidural is not an MDV and must be used only once on one patient.

16. **The correct answer is A.** Antithrombotic agents, including direct oral anticoagulants such as apixaban, are on the ISMP high-risk/high-alert medication list. Buproprion, citalopram, and aripiprazole are not considered high-risk medications.

17. **The correct answer is A.** Hydromorphone is a Schedule II medication and is not permitted refills. The other answer choices—1 refill, 5 refills in 6 months, and no restrictions on refills—are all noncompliant options for Schedule II narcotics.

18. **The correct answer is D.** Adherence can be calculated as a percentage using the total days' supply for all patient fills divided by the total days in a given period.

Adherence Percentage =

$$\frac{\text{Total Days' Supply of Patient Fills}}{\text{Total Days}} \times 100$$

If a patient filled a medication for a 30-day supply 8 times in one year, this would be 240 days of total therapy divided by 365 days of total time.

$$\frac{240 \text{ total days' supply}}{365 \text{ total days}} \times 100 = 66\%$$

19. **The correct answer is D.** International Unit (IU) can be mistaken for IV (intravenous). International Unit should always be written out and not abbreviated. U (for units) is often confused with 0. IM may be confused with IN (intranasal). TPN does not have a confused drug abbreviation.

20. **The correct answer is C.** Trailing zeroes should never be used when writing dosage forms, as they can be easily confused. This eliminates choice A (9.0 mg) and choice D (9.0 mcg). The abbreviation for milligram is mg, not mcg as shown in choice B. The correct way to write nine milligrams is 9 mg.

21. **The correct answer is C.** Set up the alligation by putting the higher strength in the top left, lower strength in the bottom left, and desired strength in the middle.

5		
	3	
1		

Now subtract the difference to find the total parts needed and place this into the top right and bottom right squares.

5		2
	3	
1		2
		4 total parts

This means we need 2 parts of the 5% and 2 parts of the 1% hydrocortisone. Adding these together equals 4 total parts (add the right-hand column).

To determine the total grams needed to make the mixture, set up a ratio proportion calculation.

For the 5% hydrocortisone:

$$\frac{2 \text{ parts}}{4 \text{ parts}} = \frac{x \text{ grams}}{100 \text{ grams}}$$

$$(2)(100) = (4)(x)$$
$$\frac{200}{4} = x$$
$$x = 50 \text{ grams}$$

50 grams of the 5% hydrocortisone is needed.

Complete the same process for the 1% hydrocortisone.

For the 1% hydrocortisone:

$$\frac{2 \text{ parts}}{4 \text{ parts}} = \frac{x \text{ grams}}{100 \text{ grams}}$$

$$(2)(100) = (4)(x)$$

$$\frac{200}{4} = x$$

$$x = 50 \text{ grams}$$

50 grams of the 1% hydrocortisone is needed.

To check your work, add up the total grams needed for each to validate that it does equal the total desired:

$$50 \text{ grams} + 50 \text{ grams} = 100 \text{ grams}.$$

22. **The correct answer is D.** HTN is the abbreviation for hypertension, or high blood pressure. Heartburn (choice A) is generally abbreviated as GERD; headache (choice B) is HA; and high cholesterol (choice C), or hypercholesterolemia, is abbreviated as HCL.

23. **The correct answer is A.** The first set of numbers in an NDC represents the labeler, which is the manufacturer, repackager, or distributor. The second and middle set of numbers of the NDC identifies the product or drug (choice B). The third set of numbers is known as the package size (choice C). A lot number (choice D) is a number assigned by a manufacturer to a specific batch of drugs produced.

24. **The correct answer is B.** Regular insulin is good for 28 days after opening. In this case, April 29 would be the BUD. April 15 (choice A) would be a 14-day stability, and May 13 (choice C) would be a 42-day stability, which are both incorrect. The insulin is good until the expiration date on the vial (choice D) if it has not yet been punctured. After puncturing, most insulins have a 28-day expiration.

25. **The correct answer is A.** This order can be found by simply multiplying the patient's BSA by the mg dose prescribed. It can also be calculated using the ratio proportion method.

$$\frac{x \text{ mg}}{1.1 \text{ m}^2} = \frac{200 \text{ mg}}{1 \text{ m}^2}$$

$$(200 \text{ mg})(1.1 \text{ m}^2) = 220 \text{ mg}$$

26. **The correct answer is C.** PPE must be worn when compounding and handling hazardous drugs, and shoe covers and gloves can help prevent exposure and additional contamination. A lab coat (choice A) may be worn but will not prevent exposure. An isolation kit (choice B) is used for patients being cared for in isolation due to respiratory or contagious disease. A radiation dosimetry badge (choice D) detects radiation levels for those working in a radiology department.

27. **The correct answer is A.** DEA Form 41 is used for destruction of controlled substances. DEA Form 106 (choice B) must be completed in the event of a theft or loss of controlled substances. DEA Form 222 (choice C) is used to order Schedule II controlled substances, and a DEA Form 224 (choice D) is used for initial registration with the DEA.

28. **The correct answer is C.** Benzonatate is an antitussive agent. It is not a decongestant, antihistamine, or expectorant.

29. **The correct answer is B.** Celebrex is available in 100 mg and 200 mg capsules. It is not available in tablet, oral solution, or IV injection form.

30. **The correct answer is B.** The first step is to calculate how many units are in one vial. A standard insulin vial is 100 units/mL and contains 10 mL:

$$\frac{x \text{ units}}{10 \text{ mL}} = \frac{100 \text{ units}}{1 \text{ mL}}$$

$$x \text{ units} = (100)(10) = 1,000 \text{ units}$$

There are 1,000 units in one insulin vial.

Next, calculate how many units the patient will be taking daily. The order is written as TID:

$$(13 \text{ units})(3) = 39 \text{ units daily}$$

Now divide the total number of units by the daily dose:

$$\frac{1,000 \text{ units}}{39 \text{ units}} = 25 \text{ days}$$

When calculating days' supply, always round your answer down to the next whole number of days. If a patient has enough for 25.64 days, this should only be considered 25 days.

31. **The correct answer is B.** A glucometer can be recommended for at-home testing to identify blood glucose levels. A coagulation analyzer (choice A) would be used to determine INR levels for patients on anticoagulation medications. A salivary assay (choice C) is often used for at-home rapid HIV screens. A pulse oximeter (choice D) can detect oxygen saturation levels.

32. **The correct answer is C.** A drug utilization review is a review of a prescription to screen for potential drug interactions, allergies, contraindications, appropriate prescribing, and compliance. Medication adherence (choice A) is defined as taking a medication as prescribed. Medication reconciliation (choice B) is the process of comparing a patient's home med list with what medications they have prescribed as an inpatient for reconciliation of dosages. Therapeutic substitution (choice D) occurs when a medication is substituted for another in the same drug class.

33. **The correct answer is A.** Metformin is a biguanide antidiabetic agent that helps stimulate insulin release. Furosemide (choice B) is a diuretic, prednisone (choice C) is a steroid, and levothyroxine (choice D) is a hormone for thyroid treatment.

34. **The correct answer is C.** A pharmacist must sign each line on a Schedule II invoice. A pharmacy technician can neither sign (choice A) nor document inventory (choice D) on Schedule II invoices. Schedule III and IV narcotics are permitted to be stored in non-controlled inventory; vault storage (choice B) is not needed.

35. **The correct answer is D.** The ISO level determines how clean the air is—the higher the level, the dirtier the air. Among the choices given, ISO class 8 is the highest level and is therefore the dirtiest.

36. **The correct answer is A.** First, multiply the patient's BSA by the mg dose prescribed. It can also be calculated using ratio proportion:

$$\frac{x \text{ mg}}{1.6 \text{ m}^2} = \frac{15 \text{ mg}}{1 \text{m}^2}$$

$$(15 \text{ mg})(1.6 \text{ m}^2) = 24 \text{ mg}$$

Now that we know the dose, we can use a dosage calculation to solve for the volume based on the medication in stock:

$$\frac{x \text{ mL}}{24 \text{ mg}} = \frac{5 \text{ mL}}{100 \text{ mg}}$$

Solve for x:

$$x = \frac{(24 \text{ mg})(5 \text{ mL})}{100 \text{ mg}}$$
$$x = 1.2 \text{ mL}$$

37. **The correct answer is D.** Schedule II controlled substances must be stored within a vault or safe in the pharmacy. If stocked at a nursing unit within an automated dispensing cabinet (ADC), it must be locked and not stored within an open matrix drawer.

38. **The correct answer is A.** Insulin syringes are used for diabetic patients for insulin administration. These syringes are 1 mL or less and are measured in both mL and units for insulin dosing. Tuberculin syringes (choice B) are small syringes that hold up to 1 mL and are used for intradermal administration of a purified protein derivative (PPD). Hypodermic syringes (choice C) are typically plastic syringes that range in size

from 3 mL to 60 mL. These syringes can also be used for oral administration. There are no ampule syringes (choice D).

39. **The correct answer is D.** Lamotrigine is an anticonvulsant indicated for the treatment of epilepsy. It is not an antifungal agent, antihistamine, or antidiabetic.

40. **The correct answer is A.** TE code A is considered therapeutically equivalent. B codes are not considered therapeutic equivalent. There are no TE codes C or D.

41. **The correct answer is A.** An injury caused by a drug is known as an adverse drug event (ADE). ADEs include adverse drug reactions, overdoses, and harm from the discontinuation of drug therapy. A near miss (choice B) is not an error and would not be included. Polypharmacy (choice C) has the potential to cause errors but is not an error. Therapeutic substitution (choice D) occurs when a medication is substituted for another in the same drug class and is not considered an error.

42. **The correct answer is B.** A provider must be registered with the DEA to prescribe a controlled substance, and this DEA number must be on the prescription. Patient allergies, pharmacy phone number, and patient medical record number do not need to be included on a prescription for controlled substances.

43. **The correct answer is A.** A prospective DUR is generally completed at insurance adjudication or submission and is electronically reviewed prior to approval. If a DUR is completed after the patient has received the medication (choice B), it is known as a retrospective DUR. Patients are not always granted refills for every prescription, so choice C would not be accurate. The pharmacist has not yet seen the order to complete the DUR when the patient is being prescribed the medication, so choice D is not possible.

44. **The correct answer is B.** Janumet is a combination drug used for diabetes treatment. It is made of metformin and sitagliptin. Glipizide, liraglutide, and glyburide are not in Janumet.

45. **The correct answer is C.** Levothyroxine has a narrow therapeutic index. Clindamycin, triamcinolone, and rosuvastatin do not have narrow therapeutic indexes.

46. **The correct answer is C.** First convert tsp to mL:

$$\frac{x \, \text{mL}}{3 \, \text{tsp}} = \frac{5 \, \text{mL}}{1 \, \text{tsp}} = \frac{(3)(5)}{1} = 15 \, \text{mL}$$

Next, determine the daily dosage. TID = 3 × a day; (15)(3) = 45 mL daily.

The patient is taking this for 7 days, so (45)(7) = 315 mL is needed.

125 mL and 250 mL would not be sufficient sizes to fill this order. The size given in choice C (360 mL) is more than what is needed but will cover the entire order and will not waste as much as the 480 mL size would.

47. **The correct answer is D.** If converting from a smaller unit to a bigger unit, such as mcg to mg, divide by 1,000 or move the decimal point to the left 3 places.

$$\frac{75}{1,000} = 0.075 \, \text{mg}$$

48. **The correct answer is D.** A CAI may also be used to compound non-hazardous products and includes the cleaning of the ante chamber next to the main compounding chamber. There is no buffer *chamber* (choice A)—only a buffer room. The HEPA filter (choice B) is certified and inspected, but should not be cleaned or sprayed with cleaner. A glove box (choice C) is another name for a CAI.

49. **The correct answer is B.** Humira is an immunosuppressive drug used to treat psoriasis and Crohn's disease. Nodular acne (choice

A) is treated with isotretinoin. Impetigo (choice C) is treated with Bactroban; athlete's foot, jock itch, and ringworm (choice D) are treated with Lotrimin or Lamisil.

50. **The correct answer is B.** Methocarbamol is the generic name of Robaxin. Carisoprodol (choice A) is the generic of Soma, chlorthalidone (choice C) is the generic of Thalitone, and brimonidine (choice D) is the generic of Alphagan.

51. **The correct answer is B.** A dispensing error can result from calculation errors, incorrect patient selection, or inappropriate refills, such as early refills. A patient prescribed a medication Q4–6HPRN could be taking the medication a maximum of 6 times daily. If 24 tablets are dispensed with 6 being taken each day, this is a 4-day supply only. Tramadol can be taken every 4 to 6 hours, so this is not a prescribing error. There is no information to indicate the patient may misuse the medication or has an allergy to tramadol.

52. **The correct answer is B.** Hydralazine is an antihypertensive agent used for high blood pressure. It is not used to treat cholesterol, diabetes, or inflammation.

53. **The correct answer is D.** Use the equation $C_1V_1 = C_2V_2$ to determine the amount needed.

$C_1 = 12$
$V_1 = x$
$C_2 = 4$
$V_2 = 1,000$

Solve for x.

$$(12)(x) = (4)(1,000)$$
$$x = \frac{(4)(1,000)}{12}$$
$$x = 33$$

333 mL of stock solution is needed.

This question also asks for quantity of diluent needed with the stock solution. This

can be found by taking the final volume and subtracting the stock volume calculated:

$$1,000 \text{ mL} - 333 \text{ mL} = 667 \text{ mL}$$

667 mL diluent is added to 333 mL stock solution to get a final volume of 1,000 mL.

54. **The correct answer is B.** A compounding aseptic containment isolator (CACI) is used for hazardous drug compounding. A CAI (choice A) and horizontal flow hood (choice C) are used for non-hazardous drug compounding. HEPA (choice D) is the type of filter in PECs.

55. **The correct answer is B.** Antibiotics that are fluoroquinolones often end in –*oxacin* (such as levofloxacin or ciprofloxacin). Steroids end in –*one* (prednisone, triamcinolone), antivirals end in –*vir* (oseltamivir, acyclovir), and antihyperlipidemics that are statins end in –*statin* (atorvastatin, rosuvastatin).

56. **The correct answer is C.** There are several questions to consider when conducting an RCA: 1) What happened? 2) What usually happens? 3) Why did it happen? 4) What can we do to prevent it from happening again? 5) What actions can be measured? It is important during this data gathering that no blame is placed or punitive action administered on the employee(s) involved. It is also important to acknowledge human error as a factor, but to look past this component and identify potential systematic, workflow, or other major issues that contributed to this event. When investigating a medication event, it is not helpful to use the outcome of the patient for evaluation, as this could create an outcome bias (e.g., determining the level of response based on whether or not the patient was harmed).

57. **The correct answer is A.** A prescription for a Schedule II controlled substance cannot be transferred to another pharmacy, even if the pharmacies are in the same chain.

58. The correct answer is C. Synergism occurs when the combined effect of two drugs is much larger or longer in duration than the sum of the two. Summation or addition (choice A) occurs when the effect of two drugs is the same as the effect each drug would have if taken individually; essentially the "sum" of taking the drugs together. Potentiation (choice B) is an interaction that causes one drug to prolong or increase the effect of another drug. Antagonism (choice D) is the interaction between two drugs in which one drug works against the other.

59. The correct answer is D. Computerized provider order entry (CPOE) helps prevent errors by eliminating manual writing of prescriptions. Through an electronic process, providers can pick the dosage that is safe, instead of writing by hand. Prescribing errors are often caused by communication failure—either through misinterpretation of handwriting, verbal orders (transcribing), or the use of ineligible or confusing abbreviations, so using confusing abbreviations (choice A) would not be safe. CPOE does not involve verbal orders (choice B). CPOE would not prevent dispensing an expired medication (choice C) as the order is placed before the drug product selection occurs.

60. The correct answer is D. The width or diameter of the needle increases as the gauge number decreases. Of the choices listed, a 30 G needle is the smallest. Smaller gauge or larger needles are chosen for solutions that are more viscous, as the solution can be withdrawn or administered more easily. Larger gauge or finer needles are used for patient administration to minimize pain during injection.

61. The correct answer is A. Within the PEC, the ISO level cannot be greater than ISO class 5. ISO classes 6, 7, and 8 would not be sufficiently clean for sterile compounding.

62. The correct answer is A. Lansoprazole is an antiulcer agent/proton pump inhibitor, and it can be used for the treatment of GERD. It is not used for high cholesterol (choice B), rhinitis (choice C), or nausea and vomiting (choice D).

63. The correct answer is D. Grapefruit juice and statins cause a drug-nutrient interaction because grapefruit juice increases the absorption of these drugs, which can cause an enhanced effect. Milk, tea, and coffee are all safe to drink while taking rosuvastatin.

64. The correct answer is B. A sublingual tablet is placed under the tongue and dissolves. A buccal tablet (choice A) is placed between the gums and the cheek and dissolves. Enteric-coated tablets (choice C) are designed to prevent dissolving in the stomach and intended to bypass the stomach and dissolve in the intestine. An effervescent tablet (choice D) is one that contains a substance, such as sodium bicarbonate, that reacts with water to give off carbon dioxide (and causes a fizz) and must be dissolved before administration.

65. The correct answer is D. Hood cleaning should be done at the beginning of every shift, every 30 minutes or before every batch, and if a spill occurs. This cleaning must be documented in a daily log. Although cleaning at the end of the day (choice A) is appropriate, it is not the only time cleaning is required. Cleaning should also be done *before* every batch—not after it is completed (choice B). Every 60 minutes (choice C) would not be frequent enough for cleaning.

66. The correct answer is B. The intradermal route is an injection into the top layer of the skin. The intra-arterial route (choice A) is an injection into an artery. The intravenous route (choice C) is an injection into the vein, while the intramuscular route (choice D) is an injection into the muscle.

67. **The correct answer is B.** *Transdermal* denotes the application of a medication through the skin, and this is typically done via a patch. The otic route (choice A) is through or in the ear. The parenteral route (choice C) refers to anything given via injection or infusion (bypasses the intestine), and an IV push (choice D) is a bolus dose of a medication given intravenously.

68. **The correct answer is C.** A graduated cylinder is a straight-sided measuring device for liquids that comes in different sizes for volume measurements. A mortar (choice A) is a bowl used with a pestle for grinding solids into powder. A weigh boat (choice B) is used for weighing powders or substances on a balance. An ointment slab (choice D) is a large, thick piece of glass (or porcelain) used for mixing when compounding ointments.

69. **The correct answer is A.** Reye's syndrome is a serious condition involving swelling in the brain and liver damage that can occur in children receiving aspirin. Stevens-Johnson syndrome (choice B) consists of a painful red or purple rash that spreads and blisters, and it is caused by allopurinol, acetaminophen, ibuprofen, penicillin, or anticonvulsants. Tendon rupture (choice C) can occur when taking a fluoroquinolone antibiotic. Tooth discoloration (choice D) can occur if tetracycline is given to a child.

70. **The correct answer is C.** An ADC is a cabinet located securely in a nursing unit for dispensing of frequently used medications. It does not dispense only IVs (choice A) and is not located in patient rooms (choice B). An ADC is not located in the pharmacy (choice D), as the pharmacy has the main stock of medications.

71. **The correct answer is C.** Garbing is completed dirtiest to cleanest, so shoe covers are donned first in the ante room. Next, a hair cover (and beard cover if needed) should be donned, along with a face mask. Following this step, hand washing should occur. A hand scrub is used after a gown has been donned, prior to donning sterile gloves.

72. **The correct answer is D.** When an ampule is opened, the glass must be broken, and the contents are then exposed to air. It should not be opened until immediately prior to use. An SDV, though used for only one dose, is not exposed to the air. An MDV is good for 28 days, and most insulin vials are as well.

73. **The correct answer is C.** Meloxicam is an NSAID, which is a drug class that requires a medication guide be dispensed. Atorvastatin, atenolol, and lisinopril do not require medication guides.

74. **The correct answer is B.** Cefdinir is an antibiotic used to treat bacterial infections. A cold is a viral infection, and the use of an antibiotic to treat any viral infection is an overuse prescribing error. Underuse (choice A) occurs when a medication that would help the disease state of the patient is inadvertently not prescribed. Misuse (choice C) occurs if a medication is prescribed that leads to unfavorable outcomes, such as when a contraindication is overlooked, and a patient has an adverse event. An administration error (choice D) occurs when a medication is administered via the wrong route, given to the wrong patient, or at the wrong time.

75. **The correct answer is D.** Benzonatate is an antitussive medication, which is used for relief of cough. It does not relieve rhinitis, congestion, or fever.

76. **The correct answer is A.** Adalimumab (Humira) is given by injection, and a side effect may be pain at the injection site. Loperamide, methylcellulose, and clonazepam are all given orally.

77. **The correct answer is D.** Monitoring errors may often include a lack of response when a patient requires a modification to the prescribed dosing. In this case, dosing modifications are often necessary when a patient has decreased renal function. If this is missed, a monitoring error has occurred. This would not be considered a prescribing error (choice A) because the original order

was correct. The correct drug was dispensed, so this would not be a dispensing error (choice B), and there was no issue in administration (choice C).

78. **The correct answer is D.** A desiccant is designed to absorb excess moisture in a stock bottle, which helps prevent deterioration of the drug. Light degradation (choice A) is prevented with amber vials or bottles. Protecting a medication from heat exposure (choice B) would involve proper storage. Physical incompatibilities (choice C) result when medications are compounded or mixed.

79. **The correct answer is A.** Ginseng can be used to boost energy, lower blood sugar, reduce cholesterol, and reduce stress. Saw palmetto can be used for BPH; valerian and melatonin can be used for insomnia. Migraines can be treated with feverfew.

80. **The correct answer is D.** Vitamin K (phytonadione) is essential for blood clotting and can be given to patients who are bleeding excessively due to the use of an anticoagulant. Vitamin A (choice A) is important for vision, vitamin D_2 (choice B) helps absorb calcium and phosphorus, and vitamin E (choice C) is an antioxidant.

81. **The correct answer is A.** Sulfa drugs can cause photosensitivity as a side effect. Bactrim is sulfamethoxazole and trimethoprim. Tegretol (choice B), Percocet (choice C), and Lantus (choice D) are all in drug classes that do not cause photosensitivity.

82. **The correct answer is D.** Spironolactone is a potassium-sparing diuretic, and this potassium-sparing effect combined with the increased potassium effect of ACE inhibitors, such as enalapril, can cause hyperkalemia. Metoprolol (choice A) is a beta blocker, verapamil (choice B) is a calcium channel blocker, and losartan (choice B) is an ARB. These classes do not have the potassium-sparing effect seen in ACE inhibitors.

83. **The correct answer is B.** To prevent dispensing errors, it is important to utilize barcode scanning technology to confirm drug product, strength, and dosage form selection. CPOE (choice A) helps prevent prescribing errors. Monitoring creatinine levels (choice C) can help prevent monitoring errors. Using the "five rights" (choice D) helps to prevent administration errors.

84. **The correct answer is C.** Carbidopa/levodopa tablets should be stored at room temperature, which is 20°C to 25°C. Choice A (2°C to 8°C) is refrigerated storage, and choice B (8°C to 15°C) is considered "cool" storage. Choice D (30°C to 40°C) would be warm storage—i.e., too warm for room temperature.

85. **The correct answer is C.** Meloxicam (Mobic) is available as 7.5 mg and 15 mg tablets. It is not available as in a capsule or cream form.

86. **The correct answer is C.** Diuretics should be taken in the morning to prevent the need to urinate at night. HMG-CoA reductase inhibitors (choice A) should be taken at nighttime due to cholesterol production occurring at night. Beta blockers (choice B) are often taken at night because fatigue is one of the side effects. Hypnotics (choice D) should always be taken at bedtime, due to their sedative properties.

87. **The correct answer is D.** Because Coumadin is used to prevent blood clots, unexpected bleeding could be a side effect if the dosing is not appropriate or a patient has a drug interaction. Vitamin K (choice A) helps clot blood, so bleeding would not be a side effect. Bactrim DS (choice B) is an antimicrobial agent, and Claritin (choice C) is an antihistamine—neither would cause bleeding as a side effect.

Answers Practice Test 2

88. **The correct answer is C.** The FDA has a reporting system for adverse and safety events known as MedWatch. This program provides a voluntary and online reporting tool to report serious adverse events or product quality concerns. It is through this database that the FDA may initiate investigations with manufacturers for potential recalls. MERP, or Medication Error Reporting Program (choice A), is similar to MedWatch, but ISMP cannot initiate recalls or make recommendations to manufacturers. AHRQ (choice B) is the Agency for Healthcare Research and Quality and reviews medication errors for potential trends in practice. An RCA (choice D) helps identify the cause of medication errors.

89. **The correct answer is A.** Trituration is the process of creating smaller particles through crushing, grinding, or pulverizing using a mortar and pestle. Levigation (choice B) is the process of combining a powder with a liquid; for example, mineral oil (for water-soluble bases) and glycerin (for oil-soluble bases). Spatulation (choice C) is a technique in which a spatula is used for mixing, usually on an ointment slab. Geometric dilution (choice D) is a method of mixing two substances of unequal quantities, starting with the smallest quantity and mixing an equal amount of the largest quantity until all the ingredients have been added.

90. **The correct answer is A.** Use the equation $C_1V_1 = C_2V_2$ to determine the amount needed.

$C_1 = 6$

$V_1 = x$

$C_2 = 2$

$V_2 = 250$

Solve for x:

$$(6)(x) = (2)(250)$$
$$x = \frac{(2)(250)}{6}$$
$$x = 83.3$$

83.3 mL of stock solution is needed.

This question also asks for quantity of diluent needed with the stock solution. This can be found by taking the final volume and subtracting the stock volume calculated:

$$250 \text{ mL} - 83.3 \text{ mL} = 166.7 \text{ mL}$$

166.7 mL diluent is added to 83.3 mL stock solution to get a final volume of 250 mL.